I'M NOT
IN THE
MOOD

ALSO BY JUDITH REICHMAN, M.D.

I'm Too Young to Get Old:
Health Care for Women After Forty

I'M NOT
IN THE
MOOD

WHAT EVERY WOMAN SHOULD KNOW
ABOUT IMPROVING HER LIBIDO

JUDITH REICHMAN, M.D.

WILLIAM MORROW AND COMPANY, INC.
NEW YORK

It is the policy of William Morrow and Company, Inc., and its imprints and affiliates, recognizing the importance of preserving what has been written, to print the books we publish on acid-free paper, and we exert our best efforts to that end.

Library of Congress Cataloging-in-Publication Data

Reichman, Judith.
I'm not in the mood : what every woman should know about improving her libido / Judith Reichman.
p.   cm.
Includes index.
ISBN 0-688-16515-X
1. Sexual desire disorders—Popular works.   2. Testosterone—Therapeutic use—Popular works.   3. Testosterone—Physiological effect—Popular works.
4. Women—Sexual behavior—Popular works.   5. Sexual excitement—Popular works.   I. Title.
RC560.S46R43   1998
613.9'54—dc21   98-28544
CIP

Printed in the United States of America

First Edition

5   6   7   8   9   10

BOOK DESIGN BY MICHAEL MENDELSOHN AT MM DESIGN 2000, INC.

www.williammorrow.com

I dedicate this book

TO MY PATIENTS

who have shared their most intimate health struggles

and victories with me.

ACKNOWLEDGMENTS

IF MY TOTAL "THANK YOU" can be converted to a pie chart, the largest portion goes to Dana Points, whose help in researching and writing this book was enormous (or, using the word my copy editor wanted to delete from the text: humongous). My literary agents (what a wonderful plural term), Maureen and Eric Lasher, enthusiastically encouraged me and my publishers to go forth and proclaim: Women should know more about their libidos. So, they definitely deserve a generous piece of my thank-you pie.

Meaghan Dowling, my editor, kept this book and me in form, on-line, and in humor. My copy editor, Lisa Wolff, also worked hard to keep me readable and grammatically correct. Thank you.

My husband, Gil Cates, read the first manuscript and gave me the best advice: "Stick to what you know and are comfortable with; you're not a sex therapist." Gil, as usual, you were right, and despite this, I love you. My friends were also wonderfully helpful; Martha Luttrell reminded me that a career is not a single shot at *People* magazine, but a thoughtful plan to fulfill a purpose and leave a message. My message remains that of women's health. Lynne Wasserman, as always, was there to encourage me, offering corrections and suggestions on the first manuscript. Susan Hyatt taught me the ABC's of sexual therapy and has helped many of my patients. Her contribution to Chapter 14 was vital. Dr. Alan Decherney studied the endocrine portions of the book and gave me something I truly appreciated—a medical blessing. Dr. Laura Schlessinger, whose common sense and wisdom has enthralled America, gave me a psychological thumbs-up and a smile. Thank you, Laura. And, although I acknowledged her amazing contribution to public awareness of women's libido issues in my prologue, I once more want to express my profound thanks to Cristina Ferrare, who spoke out, spoke up, and got me into this in the first place. Cristina, your candor, humor, and positive approach has helped all women.

I want to express my appreciation to the staff at Cedars-Sinai Medical Center library and those at UCLA who, with great seriousness, helped me get articles on topics such as stress and sex, libido-reducing diseases, and medical aphrodisiacs.

My staff, especially Ana Tabares, assisted in the medical searches and also reworked my schedule so I would have some quality writing time.

I want to acknowledge the fact that my parents and daughters never once said, "You're writing a book about *what?*" My mother's more positive comment was "Good, women need to know." My daughter informed me that I didn't have to worry, *she* was fine!

Finally, thank you to all of my patients who shared their histories and problems with me. You made me realize how important libido is to mental and physical health, as well as overall well-being.

Judith Reichman, M.D.

CONTENTS

My Prolonged Prologue   1

PART ONE
THE SEXUAL FACTS

1. The "Why" of Desire   9
2. Who's Doing It—and Not Doing It   17
3. How Hormones Rule Our Moods   23
4. "I'm Not in the Mood . . ."   37

PART TWO
THE SEVEN SEXUAL SABOTEURS

5. Psychological Issues   47
6. Couple Trouble   56
7. Medications   61
8. Diseases   73
9. Surgery, Chemotherapy and Radiation   80
10. Pain   88
11. The Seventh Saboteur: Men   94

PART THREE
THE LIBIDINOUS SOLUTIONS

12. Testosterone and Beyond:
    Our Newest Hormone Replacement Options   105

13.　More Than Hormones: Alternatives and Adjuncts　　　129

14.　Can We Talk?　　　141

A Personal Aside　　　158

Resources and Recommended Readings　　　161

Bibliography　　　168

Index　　　185

I'M NOT
IN THE
MOOD

MY PROLONGED PROLOGUE

I'VE SPENT THE LAST 25 YEARS treating women. I decided to specialize in obstetrics and gynecology because I was attracted to the drama and excitement of delivering babies and the controlled suspense of the operating room. The word *control* really defines the reason that I and my colleagues (most of whom were male) were willing to put up with sleepless nights and long, grueling days. When we stepped into the delivery room or the O.R., we became green-gowned demigods with the power to heal. Those of us who thought too much about our concomitant power to cause harm probably didn't make it through the training and switched to more contemplative specialties such as internal medicine, neurology or psychiatry.

Thousands of patients (and yes, deliveries and surgeries) later, I realized that the real power lies not in deftly wielding my scalpel or, to be more high-tech, my laser beam, but in thoughtfully listening to my patients' problems, exploring the neurological, endocrinological and psychological aspects of these issues, and then contemplating the medical solutions. But the most profound "control" is ultimately helping women understand their bodies so that they can make sense out of all the medical information, misinformation, sense and nonsense with which we are bombarded. It has been said in many ways—the computer is mightier than the knife.

We humans are unique in the animal kingdom, not just because we possess opposable thumbs or have developed what we hope is a superior intellect, but also because our sexual desire is more than a need to propagate. As women, we value sex as an expression of our affection and a means to access the pleasures of our bodies' response. We start to develop our libido in puberty, and most of us hope to maintain or even improve our sexual desire and pleasure for the rest of our lives. Keeping our libido intact through the stress of finding the right partner (amid an ever-present fear of also finding a sexually transmitted disease), and then through our decades of reproducing and child rearing, through the tedium of our daily lives and daily mates and during the hormonal loss and body changes that accompany perimenopause and menopause, is not easy. Add to this the changes in our health with age, use of medications and societal expectations, and it's clear that libido maintenance is complicated—and few medical doctors "are in" or feel comfortable helping us. All of this amounts to the philosophical reason that I have included libido care in the woman care of my patients.

There is another reason that I decided to write *I'm Not in the Mood*. Over the past five years, much of my practice has been, to put it somewhat succinctly, hormonal. I've been very interested in the changes that we undergo in our forties during perimenopause and menopause and the effect of our diminishing hormones on our sense of well-being, our health and the diseases that debilitate or kill us. But I have also been astounded at how many libido-altering events occur in even younger women. After I wrote *I'm Too Young to Get Old: Health Care for Women Over Forty*, I suddenly became the hormone maven (I would have preferred "doyenne," but apparently this appellation is reserved for those who deal with issues of art, dress and food). My patients have felt that I, in my maven capacity, would have the expertise to help them overcome diminished libido. I never publicly discuss my patients, but since Cristina Ferrare went on her

TV show and announced to the world (well, at least to the viewers of her syndicated program) that she had lost her libido and that I helped her to retrieve it, I can, with her permission, use her name.

At the age of 47, Cristina felt that her lack of sexual interest and problems in getting "jump-started" would affect her wonderful marriage. She still had regular cycles, albeit increasing PMS, and when we tested her hormones, we found that her pituitary was working just a little bit harder to try to get her ovaries to successfully put out estrogen, but that her level of testosterone was low. I suggested that she try using a 2 percent testosterone ointment to see if it helped, and what a difference it made! She raved about it on her show and contacted someone who has always been interested in empowering women—Oprah Winfrey. Oprah and her production team then did their homework. They asked women with libido problems to sign onto the Internet and talk to them. The response was overwhelming and, as a result, I found myself with Cristina on Oprah's show, where we opened a sexual Pandora's box. On the plane home from Chicago, I had a sudden panic attack: What would this newfound connection with sex do to my reputation as a gynecologist? How would it affect the books I planned to write on women's health? I called my husband from the airplane phone and decried in a very loud voice (obviously volume is necessary from 30,000 feet) that I was now destined to become the doctor for women who couldn't come! The gentleman sitting next to me showed major concern and asked if he could get me a drink!

When I got home, the phones certainly did ring. As a matter of fact, the operators at Cedars-Sinai Medical Center, where I practice, told us that they couldn't handle other doctors' calls for several days because their lines were too swamped. Hundreds of women asked for appointments, but I've been able to see only a few. Their stories, like the ones related by women on the *Oprah Winfrey Show*, were wrenching and often similar. They were confronted with denial, dismissal and discouragement by the doctors they saw in an effort to seek medical help. Here are a few sample stories:

- A 46-year-old woman, married for 20 years, had a severe decline in her libido over the past two years. When she asked her doctor's advice, she was told to find a new partner to increase the spice of sex.
- A young mother with two children who was still breast-feeding her younger child felt her marriage was in jeopardy because at the end of the day, the only thing she wanted to do was put her head on a pillow and go to sleep. Her doctor's advice was to use a lubricant and "grin and bear it."
- A 34-year-old woman who underwent a hysterectomy and removal of both ovaries for cancer was told she was lucky to be alive and that her lack of libido was trivial.
- A 50-year-old woman who had just started hormone replacement therapy confided in her doctor that she missed her past feelings of sexuality. She was told that this was part of getting older. She was already on estrogen; nothing else could be done and she should get used to it.

I, by now, had started to think that it was time to write about libido and begin to set the record straight. But the final push (note I've refrained from using the word *thrust*) came once more from Oprah's power and the doctors who showed up for another libido segment to basically "put down" the entire issue and some of the therapies we had offered. There was a sudden blitz of testosterone-bashing. Dr. Nancy Snyderman, medical correspondent for *Good Morning America*, stated that any testosterone cream would be immediately absorbed into the bloodstream and have dire effects. Why, she asked, would we ever want to use it? After all, it's our estrogen that protects our hearts and makes us different from men. She then went on to comment that our brain was our most important sex organ and that if we had problems "we should watch a dirty movie."

Another physician stated that any amount of testosterone would cause us to have a heart attack. Even my colleague from the *Today* show, Dr. Bob Arnot, expressed anxiety over the use of testosterone and the risk of heart disease. His example was that estrogen seemed great at first, but we now know that long-term use can be dangerous, causing breast cancer. Well, I have to respectfully disagree. We don't know—we're still weighing the possible increase in risk of breast cancer against the many health benefits of estrogen replacement. Neither hormone deserves to be summarily dismissed or maligned.

That cinched it. My reservations about joining Dr. Ruth Westheimer in the pantheon of sex therapists paled next to my dismay at allowing misinformation about our hormones, health and libido to prevail. I'm not offering a "one therapy fits all" cure. As I told my editor, who wanted the word *cure* in the title of this book, there are few cures in medicine with the exception of antibiotics, but there *is* help and improvement.

So let's look at our libido and sexuality from a medical point of view. Are we reaching our biological sexual potential, and if not, why not? How do our hormones control our sense of well-being, spark our passion, or fuel our sexual response? If we're not in the mood or can't respond to the mood, is it because we're low on the right hormones, or high on the wrong ones? Can we separate the deep psychological and social issues that shape our sexuality from the physical aspects of our bodies? In other words, can our brains be separated from our glands?

We've learned to medicate our way to better or, at least, easier living, but what has this done to our sexual lives? Which of the many over-the-counter or prescription drugs that we take ultimately turn us off? For those of us who have had cancer, does the cure necessarily result in a loss—of our libido or sexual response? One third of us have had or will undergo a hysterectomy. Does this or other surgeries affect our sexual function?

For most of us, sex is as good as the availability, desirability and potency of our partners. The last factor has been prominently addressed (or should I say *raised?*) by the drug Viagra. How will that affect us? And, by the way, can we take this medication?

I've scanned the literature to pose these questions and tried to find the answers, and I have "come up" with some solutions. There is a role for hormones—yes, even the much-maligned testosterone. It's not a magic bullet, and it should be used only when appropriate and under careful medical supervision. There are also other pro-sexual therapies that we can consider, but most of us can't do this on our own. We need to talk to our partners, our doctors or even appropriate therapists. I've tried to make the search for sexual information and therapy easy and accessible. Denial, embarrassment and shame are not desirable female attributes.

We all possess a need for intimacy and sexual expression. Here are medical answers that will help us get in the mood for this essential aspect of our lives, well-being and health.

PART ONE

THE
SEXUAL FACTS

CHAPTER ONE

THE "WHY" OF DESIRE

W HAT MAKES US WANT SEX? Is it only that we, like other animals, possess a primitive need to mate and propagate? Or are our sexual urges, like ourselves, more highly evolved? What is libido? Is it purely physical attraction, or is it fed by fantasy—those wonderful day (and night) dreams that make us feel aroused? What prompts us to engage in sexual stimulation? Must we have a partner? Need it be someone we know, or can it be an idealized model in formal attire at the Academy Awards or, better yet, in a bathing suit in the Bahamas?

The answer to these questions is yes . . . yes . . . and, oh yes! (And we haven't even gotten to the subject of orgasm.) Libido is a product of our psychological, social *and* physical development. It is where our bodies meet up with our culture, our instincts—and what our parents and teachers taught us.

All these libidinous issues have kept the psychologists and sociologists very busy. But what about the biologists? Our sexual urges start in ancient centers in our brain that are fundamental to the propagation of our species. Hidden in the recesses of our hypothalamus and limbic system are intricate hormone receptors that bind with and are turned on by estrogen, progesterone, male hormones, prolactin, endorphins and possibly pheromones. These and our brain cells don't get their information just from hormones but also from chemicals called neurotransmitters, which form our link with the outside world.

Alas, our need for sex is not as simple as our need for chocolate (although the latter is sometimes as important to our mood and sense of well-being). We can't forget that our sexual appetite, like our premenstrual cocoa craving, is driven by fluctuations of our hormones. And if they neither fluctuate nor are present, our sexual brain centers are deadened and our appetites are dulled.

OUR STAGES OF SEXUAL RESPONSE

Most of us would consider libido to be synonymous with desire, but this is just part of the larger picture of sexual response. When scientists do their necessary categorization of sexuality (and let's face it, you can't have science without charts, tables and categories), they talk about sex in terms of stages: desire, arousal and orgasm (climax), followed by physical and mental relaxation, also known as resolution. So in the interest of science, let's follow this outline.

DESIRE

Desire, or at least an overwhelming interest in sex, begins at puberty. This transition is governed by our hormones, and we'll explore it in greater detail in Chapter 3. Suffice it to say that sweet little girls become boy-crazed adolescents thanks to the same male hormones that convert little boys (and politicians) into sexually driven beings. Even in the midst of this pubescent male-hormone surge, psychological factors play a critical role. Studies have shown that whether girls act on their fantasies and begin to have intercourse depends on their peer group—who they hang out with—and their religious background. (Unfortunately for parents, their influence is less important.)

AROUSAL

Aside from that wonderful sense of warmth, contentment and eagerness to get on with it that lets us know we're aroused, there are anatomic changes that cause our bodies to be receptive to sex.

Vasocongestion is a swelling of the blood vessels in our lower genitalia that results in increased blood flow to the labia, clitoris and vagina. This brings extra oxygen and nutrients to these arousal-essential areas on an as-needed basis. The latest word from the research front is that this engorgement may be due to a substance called vasoactive intestinal peptide (VIP). Our body's highest concentration of this protein is in the genital tract, and especially in the cervix. When VIP is injected intravenously, it has been found to cause a surge of blood to vaginal tissues, but only if estrogen is present. (I'm fantasizing here, but perhaps one day a VIP cream will be our starter aphrodisiac.)

The blood trapped in the dense network of vessels supplying the vagina, vulva and clitoris has no place to go, and the result is *swelling* and an increase in vaginal temperature, another stage that scientists have found necessary to delineate. Vasocongestion and swelling aren't limited to areas below the waist but can occur in our nipples and areola as well. In fact, increased blood flow to tiny vessels near the surface of our skin can cause a total-body flush that in the wrong light looks like measles and is known as a *sexual rash*.

Our vagina is naturally moist and we don't require sex to prevent it from becoming a desert environment. In its resting state, the walls of the vagina are collapsed, but they don't stick together because they are coated with a thin layer of fluid composed of secretions from our entire genital tract: fluid from the fallopian tubes, "old" cells shed by the cervix and vagina and uterine and cervical secretions. During arousal, when blood surges to this area, clear fluid, or plasma, from the engorged vessels is pushed into the vagina and what was minimal moisture now becomes lush irrigation. This is *lubrication*, our natural friction protection.

ORGASM

This is considered the peak of our sexual pleasure (not that everything leading up to this was exactly below sea level). From a physiological point of view, this phenomenal event is associated with rhythmic contractions of muscles around and in the vagina and reproductive organs, as well as an increase in breathing and heart rate. Little data exists on the biology of the female orgasm, despite the fact that researchers have been going at it since the 1950s. In order to document these contractions, the "masters" of sex (a gender-challenged appellation), William H. Masters and Virginia E. Johnson, observed and recorded more than 14,000 sex acts! They and the anatomists figured out that these contractions occur in two types of muscle, smooth and striated, that surround the anus and continue up along the sides of the vagina to the pelvis and lower abdomen. Both voluntary and involuntary contractions of these muscles enhance our arousal and enable us to climax.

Orgasm involves more than just our genitalia, and researchers justifiably went looking for a center for orgasm in the brain. They tried to record brain waves during "the act" and found that there were localized spikes of activity in an area called the thalamus. Unfortunately, their subjects all had mental disorders, so the findings are questionable. Do brain waves during orgasm in a mentally ill person differ from those of someone who is "normal"? Nobody knows. But no one is questioning that the brain is somehow involved in our sexual response.

Why do women have orgasms? Many would argue that we don't need a reason, but that doesn't satisfy medical science. So as usual, multiple theories have been expounded. I relate them without comment. Orgasm . . .

- is our reward for the danger of intercourse, with its possibility of pregnancy.

- is our signal that sex is over.
- permits relaxation of muscles in the pelvis that restores the vagina to its resting position and allows the cervix to touch the sperm-containing fluid in the vaginal apex.
- induces lassitude so that we remain in a supine position, allowing the sperm deposited in the vagina easy access to the cervix and ultimately the egg.
- triggers pelvic and uterine contractions that help pull sperm into the uterus (a phenomenon inelegantly known as "uterine insuck").
- serves as shock therapy to the brain, which results in calm and relaxation.
- is the ultimate physical union shared with a partner.
- is hard to achieve but worth striving for. (According to *The Hite Report*, only 30 to 50 percent of women experience orgasm with straightforward intercourse.)

RESOLUTION

The final phase of sexual response occurs when our body returns to its resting, nonaroused-but-content state. Our muscles relax; some of the vaginal fluid is absorbed by our lymph system and the swelling in the clitoris, vulva and vagina abates. This cool-down may be accompanied by a fine perspiration that, according to the principles of physics and evaporation, helps lower our body temperature. Some women are capable of being restimulated back to orgasm before completing the resolution phase. Ever since these "multiorgasmic" women were first described by researchers, we have proudly proclaimed our physical sexual superiority over men, most of whom need more time out to recover after orgasm and ejaculation.

THE ANATOMY OF SEX

I am going to spare you the usual illustrations or suggestions that you use magnifying mirrors for self-examination. However, in order to understand how our body responds during sex, we need some knowledge of what is "down there."

THE CLITORIS

This is our equivalent of the penis, but from a biological point of view it is more evolved because the urethra doesn't run through it (why mix urine with pleasure?). It is valid to draw this parallel because these organs develop in the embryo from the same male-hormone-sensitive tissue. When this erectile tissue is exposed to androgens secreted by the developing testes in the male fetus, it becomes a penis. When it isn't, it evolves into a clitoris. The extremely dense network of blood vessels and nerves in the clitoris make it supersensitive, and for most women this is the most critical area for sexual stimulation.

The thinner portion of the labia, or lips (the labia minora), come together and attach to form a hood, or *prepuce,* at the top of the clitoris. This protects it from regular, nonsexual wear and tear. During intercourse or stimulation, the hood may retract as the clitoris swells, presenting a larger sensitive surface.

THE VAGINA

In contrast to the exquisitely sensitive clitoral area, the vagina has few nerve endings so that light touch is almost imperceptible. In order to stimulate the nerves and muscles of this area, strong, deep pressure is necessary. This explains why vaginal stimulation is one-third as likely as clitoral stimulation to result in orgasm. It also touches upon the clitoral versus vaginal orgasm controversy. Many, if not most, women require clitoral stimulation to achieve orgasm, but there is no difference once we get there. Vaginal and clitoral orgasms are the same.

THE G SPOT

Having dismissed the vagina as a poor source of erotic arousal, we have to make an exception for an area under the pubic bone that is approximately one inch from the vaginal opening. This is the G spot, named after Ernst Gräfenberg, a male researcher who in 1944 reported that this area became swollen on stimulation and continued pressure, and that the feeling generated from this swelling could lead to orgasm. Geographically, this area was completely overlooked until is was rediscovered by Alice Ladas in 1982 (talk about expeditions!) and given the sexy appellation "G spot." The exact area has not been anatomically pinpointed, but it is somewhere around the opening of the bladder, perhaps in the adjacent periurethral glands. Whether or not we're believers in the G spot, it appears that there is an area in the front wall of the vagina that is supersensitive to deep stimulation. Because of the scientists' need to correlate our anatomy with men's, the G spot has also been called the "female prostate." Fluid may be present in this area during orgasm, but we're not sure if it comes from the glands or is simply escaped urine.

THE UTERUS

During arousal and excitement, the uterus may become engorged and may even increase in volume. You might wonder what methods were used to ascertain this. Wonder no more. Masters and Johnson reported that they actually palpitated the uterus before and after arousal and felt it increase in size by 50 to 75 percent. Subsequent studies using more sophisticated methods such as ultrasound simply have not been done to prove or disprove our sexual uterine growth. Masters and Johnson also found that the uterus contracted during orgasm, but again this hasn't been confirmed using reliable methods. Some women do perceive contractions, and say that they feel like cramps.

THE BRAIN

We have been told that the brain is our biggest sexual organ; hence its inclusion in this section. In normal circumstances sexual response requires messages from both the brain and the stimulated genitals. The brain's signals can be brought about by sight, smell, sound and fantasy. These are processed in deep, primitive areas called the orgasm center. During masturbation, orgasm is greatly facilitated by using sexual fantasies. But can fantasy alone (e.g., just the power of the brain) trigger orgasm without any input from below? Masters and Johnson reported it could, as did Alfred C. Kinsey of the famed Kinsey Institute. *The Story of O* told us it was possible. There have also been studies showing that orgasms can occur in paraplegic women who have no feelings or nerve impulses from the genitalia.

Arousal may be even more brain-based than orgasm. Women, like men, have wet dreams: proof of a physical response prompted by our deep, or REM, sleep. But this is not common, and it would appear that for most of us, the threshold for stimulation of the brain is so high that it is difficult to achieve sexual fulfillment on brainpower alone.

CHAPTER TWO

WHO'S DOING IT—AND NOT DOING IT

WHENEVER I DISCUSS SEX with my patients or friends, the prevailing concern is, "What's normal and how do I match up?" Society, scientists and the media have an irresistible need to quantify and staticize our lives. But do we really live that way? I have two—not 2.3—children. (I also have four stepchildren, so I'm way over budget.) I do not watch three hours and 46 minutes of television a day. I don't sleep eight hours a night (I wish I could). Nor do I measure out and consume the recommended 25 to 30 milligrams of fiber.

"Normal" shouldn't be used to make statistical comparisons about sex. What is important is that we establish a norm of frequency, quality and intimacy that fulfills our individual emotional and physical needs. Having given this disclaimer, I will now proceed to review the sex stats that are out there. The following figures are averages (a term I dislike almost as much as "norm") taken from two of our country's latest and best sex surveys, *The Janus Report on Sexual Behavior* (1993), which surveyed 1,418 women, and the *National Health and Social Life Survey* (1994), which surveyed 1,900 women.

HOW OFTEN ARE WE HAVING SEX?

This has been shown to vary according to many factors. As you look at the numbers, remember that frequency of intercourse may not accurately reflect the status of our libido and sexuality.

INTERCOURSE THROUGH THE AGES

	PERCENTAGE OF WOMEN		
AGE	2+ TIMES/WEEK	WEEKLY	RARELY
18 to 26	41–46	32	16–17
27 to 39	43–49	22–37	12–13
40 to 50	25–39	29–44	16–21
51 to 64	14–32	33–35	22–27
65+*	41	33	22

*Janus report only; sadly, women over 64 were not included in the other study.

INTERCOURSE: MARRIED VS. UNMARRIED

	PERCENTAGE OF WOMEN		
	2+ TIMES/WEEK	FEW TIMES/MONTH	FEW TIMES/YEAR	NEVER
Married	39	47	12	3
Cohabitating	56	35	8	1
Noncohabitating	20	24	23	32

Source: *National Health and Social Life Survey.*

ORGASM

This tabulation may have more significance vis-à-vis our libido than frequency of sex. We may agree to have intercourse in order to please our partner, conform to societal expectations or fill an emotional void. That doesn't mean we are either enjoying it or having orgasms. If we look at the numbers, it becomes apparent that orgasm is not an automatic purview of the young. Older women have learned to do it and have it better. Women between the ages of 40 and 50, for example, are considerably more likely to experience frequent orgasm than their counterparts ages 18 to 26. Orgasm is our reward for wrinkles and cellulite!

ORGASM WITH A PARTNER

	PERCENTAGE OF WOMEN			
AGE	FREQUENTLY	SOMETIMES	RARELY	NEVER
18 to 26	57–61	22–26	5–8	8–13
27 to 39	67–71	18–22	4–9	5–6
40 to 50	66–78	16–22	4–7	2–5
51 to 64	65–73	20–22	5–10	2–3
65+*	50	37	4	9

*Janus report only.

MASTURBATION

If we don't have a partner, the only way we can express or fulfill our libido is through masturbation. But even when a partner is available, women masturbate. In fact, according to the *National Health and Social Life Survey*, married women do it more often than single women.

In addition, women are more likely than men to achieve orgasm with masturbation than with intercourse. At least one survey has shown a gender difference in the onset of masturbation. We start later and often don't begin to masturbate until after we've started to have intercourse.

There is a huge variability in the reported statistics on masturbation, perhaps as a result of the way women were questioned or because of their reservations about owning up to this form of sexual arousal. Remember the response when Joycelyn Elders, M.D., our former U.S. Surgeon General, discussed masturbation? She was fired!

MASTURBATION

	PERCENTAGE OF WOMEN		
AGE	1X/WEEK OR MORE	OCCASIONALLY	NEVER
18 to 26	9–18	8–25	44–69
27 to 39	9–30	17–35	20–55
40 to 50	8–30	17–34	16–58
51 to 64	2–20	16–19	30–79
65+*	4	23	35

*Janus report only.

It's fascinating to look at other behaviors that affect our sexual activity. In 1998, the National Opinion Research Center in Chicago published a surprising finding: People who work more than 60 hours per week are about 10 percent more sexually active than those with less time-demanding jobs. Other groups in the study who had higher than "average" sexual activity included smokers, jazz fans, gun owners and those who drink alcohol. People who engaged in both smoking and drinking had sex more than twice as often as those who did neither. I remain unconvinced by (and unhappy with) this statistic; Please see Chapter 7 for details on how smoking and drinking can undermine your sex life.

Another recent newsmaking study reported that people with the most schooling have the least sex. Those with a partial college education averaged 62 sexual encounters per year. Those who completed college had sex 56 times a year, while graduate students and those with professional degrees had sex only 50 times a year, making them the least active group in the population. As a physician who has spent half my life pursuing graduate education, I would argue that perhaps it's not the schooling but the subsequent stress and career demands— as well as the problem of finding an appropriately educated mate— that impairs our sex life.

Race and religion appeared to have little effect on fantasy, frequency of sex and satisfaction in most surveys. Politics, however, did enter the sexual arena in places other than Washington. According to the Janus survey, 56 percent of ultraconservatives versus only 25 percent of ultraliberals felt that they were having "more" or "much more" sexual activity than three years ago. Since this study was completed in 1992, we have to assume that the ultraconservatives were still striving to gain a majority and may have channeled their unfulfilled energies into sexual pursuits. When it came to fantasy, the liberals did better. Thirty-three percent felt that to successfully function they fantasized "much" or "very much," whereas only 16 percent of ultraconservatives followed their dreams. Finally, I have to include one more study that looked at extramarital affairs: 23 percent of ultraconservatives were found to engage in the aforementioned activity "often" or "on an ongoing basis"; among ultraliberals this number dwindled to 16 percent.

Putting aside poking fun at politicians, I want to leave you with this: The media, with its many surveys, statistics and charts, has the ability to make us feel inadequate, below average or just plain abnormal. Some of us may be perfectly content with our sex life, yet when we study the numbers we suddenly realize we're not getting enough. Others may look at these figures and calculate that we're "fine," but wait—something is missing. Having sex by the numbers is not enough. So let's go beyond graphs and pie charts in order to understand our sexual potential, function and, yes, dysfunction.

CHAPTER THREE

HOW HORMONES RULE OUR MOODS

THE 1990s HAS BEEN A DECADE of heightened hormonal awareness for women. The topic of hormone replacement therapy with estrogen and progesterone has been both a media- and women's-luncheon favorite. Yet a recent study conducted by researchers at Yale University School of Medicine found that although 98 percent of women believe estrogen is a natural hormone and 67 percent were willing to accept progesterone as natural, only 46 percent acknowledged that testosterone, a male hormone, might be natural in women. The rest must have felt it was reserved for men.

The irony is that all of our estrogen is produced from male hormones, including testosterone. Does that mean we need male hormones in order to become who we are, the biochemical equivalent of Adam's rib? I prefer to think that women's bodies are the ultimate in evolutionary progress and that testosterone becomes estrogen in its search for a higher existence. Let's look at the hormonal surroundings in which our sexuality develops.

HORMONES THAT SHAPE OUR DEVELOPMENT

We all start out as an undifferentiated blob of cells. The blob that contains XY chromosomes develops testes, which then go on to produce testosterone, while in the absence of the testosterone produced by the testes the blob with XX chromosomes takes on the sex characteristics of a female. (XY embryos that fail to recognize their own testosterone develop as females, a condition known as testicular feminization.)

Male hormones reemerge as a defining substance in our lives at puberty, when their increased production sets off this momentous event. Before there is woman, there is a developing adolescent, and before there is menarche (the first period) there is adrenarche, when the adrenal glands mature and step up production of male hormones. Between the ages of 8 and 10, sweet young girls begin to perspire, exude body odor and grow pubic and underarm hair. This is also the time when they develop an unfounded (according to their parents) interest in the opposite sex. This is not due to the feminizing properties of estrogen, but to the libido power of male hormones.

Only in the next year or two does estrogen production in the ovaries emerge, causing another emergence: that of breasts, vulvar development and changes in the vaginal lining. The inner walls of the vagina mature from a thin, smooth, nonelastic surface to a ridged distensible one producing lubrication and discharge. Estrogen also determines skeletal formation (and our wider hips), fat distribution (our hips again) and weight gain. Most girls put on 20 to 30 pounds as a result of this sudden estrogen enhancement.

During this developmental stage another important hormone is surging: growth hormone. A girl's height increases two to three inches a year until she gets her first period. Finally, as the ovaries mature and successfully produce estrogen, there is a special signal to the brain via the hypothalamus and pituitary that causes the ovary to release an egg and produce progesterone.

This is the hormonal cycle that defines our reproductive lives. During the first two weeks, as the egg develops in its compartment (the *follicle*) estrogen is produced, which causes a buildup of the uterine lining (*endometrium*). The central orchestration for this process comes from the brain, which produces follicle stimulating hormone (FSH). Once estrogen levels surge, the brain secretes luteinizing hormone (LH), which directs the follicle to release the egg (*ovulation*). The capsule that remains once the egg has been released is called a *corpus luteum*, and it produces estrogen and progesterone. The function of progesterone is to build up the uterine lining in preparation for possible implantation of a fertilized egg. In the absence of fertilization and pregnancy, the corpus luteum dies two weeks after its formation. Now all hormonal bets are off, and there is a precipitous fall in both estrogen and progesterone. The uterine lining loses its hormonal support and sheds. This is our menstrual period.

Where does male hormone fit into this picture? The explanation is not simple, but neither is puberty, endocrinology or anything having to do with our bodies. Four central organs—not to mention our skin, fat and muscle—are involved: The brain produces hormones that control the production of our male hormones in our adrenal glands and ovaries. Under its direction our adrenals produce 25 percent of our total testosterone, as well as androstendione and dehydroepiandrosterone (DHEA). These are weaker androgens that can be converted into testosterone, which is why they are also known as prohormones. Androstendione is one-tenth as potent as testosterone, DHEA one one-hundredth, and another form of DHEA, DHEA-sulfate (DHEAS), is one one-thousandth as strong. To complicate matters, each of these hormones can also be converted into estrogen. The result is a massive pool of androgens from which our body can draw the hormones it needs.

Meanwhile, back at the ovary, more testosterone is being produced, accounting for another 25 percent of the total pool. This production peaks just before ovulation, when the ovary is stimulated by FSH. But the activated follicle is not solely responsible for ovarian male hormone production. Some comes from surrounding cells that form the matrix, or body, of the ovary. These cells are urged to become androgen producers by LH. The ovary, like the adrenal, also produces the prohormone androstendione and a very small amount of DHEA.

If our math is correct, we've accounted for 50 percent of our testosterone. Where does the rest come from? Here is where our fat, skin and muscle play their part, converting the prohormones produced by the adrenal and ovary into testosterone.

With all this male hormone circulating in the body, why aren't women more like men? The principal reason is that even though our adrenals and ovaries are potent male hormone producers, their collective effort gives us only one-tenth the amount of testosterone produced by the male testes. But there is more: In order for testosterone to work on testosterone-sensitive cells present in our skin, hair follicles, muscles, bones, brain, nipples and clitoris (with ongoing research, this list may turn out to include most of the cells in our body), it has to be converted to a more potent form, dehydrotestosterone (DHT). Masculinization of these testosterone-sensitive tissues is dictated by the presence (or absence) of the enzyme 5-alpha-reductase, which converts testosterone to DHT. Those of us who complain of excess body hair growth may have higher levels of this enzyme or make slightly more testosterone which is presented to and efficiently converted by this enzyme to DHT.

The second limiting factor of testosterone's effect on our body is that very little of the hormone is allowed to roam free. The vast majority is bound up and rendered virtually powerless by one of two proteins, albumin (whose bonds are fairly weak) and sex hormone binding globulin (SHBG), which latches on to testosterone for dear life. The end result is that only 1 percent of the potent male hormone, testosterone, is free, 4 percent of DHEA is unbound, and 7 percent of androstendione is out there on its own. So when we consider and measure levels of male hormone with blood tests, the only thing that counts is that portion that is free.

Testosterone, like men, wants to rule. Since the only way it can do this is by undermining SHBG's power, it limits the production of SHBG in the liver. Estrogen fights back, increasing SHBG production. One would think that because estrogen is also bound by SHBG, this is self-defeating. But here's the trump: SHBG attaches to testosterone three times more readily and strongly than it does to estrogen. So when the two are out there in competition, it's the male hormone that, like Samson, is bound, shorn and rendered less potent.

So now that we're hormone experts, let's see what they do for our libido.

HOW HORMONES AFFECT OUR LIBIDO

DURING PUBERTY

Although we need estrogen for comfort (i.e., lubrication) during sex, we also need fairly constant amounts of male hormone in order to feel desire and have a biological sexual response. The first inkling of what we call libido is directly connected to our production of male hormones. Testosterone causes our nipples and clitoris to become sensitive, stimulates our fantasies, masturbation and, of course, sparks our interest in the opposite sex. A study of 200 postpubertal girls showed that the major predictor of their first coital experience (a clinical way of saying intercourse) was the rise in their testosterone level. The single factor that appeared to block this effect was frequent attendance at religious services. (God is more powerful than testosterone!)

As awesome as this androgen effect is on girls, it appears to provide an even more powerful jolt to boys, possibly because they have a 10- to 20-fold increase in male hormone, whereas we have a comparatively modest doubling.

OVER THE MENSTRUAL CYCLE

Testosterone has been found to peak slightly just prior to ovulation. One would think nature would engineer it so that this higher level would spark our desire for intercourse and increase our chances of pregnancy when we're most fertile. However, most studies have had difficulty pairing cyclical fluctuations of testosterone with desire. Libido maintenance is probably dependent on steady amounts of testosterone and even if a small increase occurs, it won't make us feel sexier.

Having said this, I know from my clinical practice that significant PMS affects libido. The last thing most women want to do when they're depressed, bloated, feeling fat and having cramps is have sex. We know that depression is a major libido saboteur (see Chapter 5), and 7 percent of women suffer from premenstrual dysphoric disorder, in which depression can be severe.

DURING PREGNANCY

Our libido and sexual activity may increase, decrease or carry on as usual during pregnancy, though most studies find a decline in the third trimester. None of the changes has been related to hormone levels, so we can conclude that when estrogen and progesterone are produced in enormous amounts, as they are during pregnancy, they are irrelevant to our sexual behavior. Studies have shown that overall, sexual satisfaction is correlated with feeling happy about being pregnant and feeling attractive despite an expanding abdomen.

AFTER DELIVERY

Before "post" there is "partum": delivery of the baby. And if we have this baby vaginally we may have an episiotomy. It generally takes three to six weeks for complete healing, and during this time the very thought of intercourse is discomforting. Pain or the anticipation of pain has been shown to be one of the major saboteurs of sexual desire. Even after the episiotomy heals, a small percentage of women have localized tenderness. This may be due to the formation of a neuroma, or bundle of nerves that is so exquisitely sensitive that penetration or even slight touch can cause searing knife-like pain. For some women, the issue of healing isn't physical but psychological. If clinical postpartum depression occurs, as it does in 10 percent of women, it generally includes a lack of libido. Finally, there is the stress of a crying, demanding infant, sleep deprivation, our need as new mothers to evaluate our role in life and our partner's response to all of the above.

What about breast-feeding? We know very little about androgens in lactating women, but we do know that when we're breast-feeding we produce high levels of prolactin, which stimulates production of milk. But prolactin does more than make milk. It inhibits ovulation (which is why we don't get our periods for a long time while breast-feeding), lowers estrogen production and has been shown to depress libido. (An interesting aside: Men with elevated prolactin levels lose desire and become impotent.)

Contrary to what we might expect, Masters and Johnson found that the libido of nursing mothers rebounded more quickly in the postpartum period than did that of non-nursing mothers, but that the nursing moms' genital response was weak. (The desire was there, but the act was difficult.) Decades ago, when these studies were done, women who chose to nurse may have been more comfortable with their bodies and thus have had more positive attitudes toward sex than women who bottle-fed babies. But today, many clinicians, including myself, find it is common for women to report marked loss of sexual interest while breast-feeding. The reasons are painfully clear: When a woman breast-feeds, her postpartum drop in estrogen persists for months, and as a result the vaginal lining becomes thin and dry, much as it does during menopause. Intercourse is uncomfortable or hurts. My own Darwinian (or can I say "Reichmanian?") explanation is that evolution has conditioned our postpartum libido to remain depressed because we need to devote our energy and attention to our current progeny. We don't need the distraction of sex or the possibility of another pregnancy before we are ready.

IN PERIMENOPAUSE

Menopause does not start with a bang. It is the final whimper after a long process of ovarian follicular exhaustion. We begin puberty with about 400,000 follicles and even though only one produces a fertilizable egg each month, thousands that don't even get to this egg-producing point die. This rate of attrition dictates that eventually we will use up our follicles and our source of estrogen will disappear.

Our forties coincide with a period of follicular dwindling. Our hormones fluctuate, and our total estrogen level can decrease. We begin to have irregular cycles, increasing PMS, hot flashes, vaginal dryness, sleep disturbances and mood swings. These symptoms have ensured that estrogen gets all the attention when it comes to perimenopause. Recent evidence, however, indicates that during this transition there also may be a total or midcycle dip in our ovarian production of testosterone. We're rehearsing for menopause.

If we want to be semantically correct, we are perimenopausal when our previously normal cycles become irregular and we develop any one of the above-mentioned symptoms. The average age of perimenopause is 47.5 and the average duration of this transition is 3.8 years. Ninety percent of us will experience it, while 10 percent of us suddenly stop having our periods with nary a warning sign nor symptom. Smokers go through both perimenopause and menopause an average of 1.8 years earlier than nonsmokers.

These hormonal shifts are not unique to our ovaries. As we age, so do our adrenal glands, and by the time we reach 40, they are secreting half the male hormones that they produced when we were 20. For many of us this is a nonevent, because we are still producing enough testosterone for libido maintenance. Additionally, as our estrogen levels diminish in our forties, so does our level of SHBG. So even as our total testosterone level falls, the amount of free testosterone circulating in our blood remains relatively unchanged. There are, or course, exceptions. Some of us continue to maintain good estrogen and SHBG production, while our adrenals just don't keep up. As a result, our free testosterone levels decrease, and so does our libido and sexual response.

The combined changes in ovarian and adrenal testosterone production may be as clinically significant as any shifting hormone levels that occur later in life. Research shows that approximately one-third of women experience loss of libido during perimenopause, and the number reaches 40 percent in menopause.

IN MENOPAUSE

Even the most health-conscious women (and many of their physicians) wait for the advent of menopause to discuss, test or treat hormonal issues. And in this drama, the "tragedy" of estrogen's demise takes center stage. But before we critique the play, let's review estrogen's role in this transition and what it does to our sexual health.

Since the follicles in our ovaries have been our chief source of estrogen, once they're totally depleted, we lose 80 to 90 percent of our supply (the loss is not total because our fat cells and muscle are converting a small portion of male hormone to a weak estrogen). The lower part of our genital tract needs estrogen, and when we lose it we undergo "starvation involution." The first thing to go is vaginal fluid secretion, and the vagina fails to lubricate properly during sexual arousal and intercourse. (The vagina is so sensitive to estrogen that this change often occurs in women in their early forties.) This dry zone can be blamed on diminished blood flow to the vagina, fewer cells lining its walls, less mucus production from the cervix and less fluid coming from the uterine cavity. The vaginal walls also smooth out, becoming thinner and less elastic. The surface is now easily traumatized by intercourse, and if we're not sexually active, scar tissue can form between surfaces that touch one another. This is not a co-ital-friendly change and, for the majority of women, it will result in discomfort with intercourse (dyspareunia). Pain with sex is the second most common complaint (after hot flashes) that causes meno-pausal women to visit their gynecologist. Thirty to 40 percent of menopausal women will develop dyspareunia if they do not use estro-gen therapy.

Because of reduced blood flow to the vagina, there is less engorge-ment of the tissues during arousal. This can interfere with stimulation and orgasm. As estrogen levels decline, some women develop a type of nerve apathy. They have numbness and aversion to touch. Ca-resses may become unpleasant or even irritating. Estrogen has one other effect down under: It promotes muscle tone, and in its absence our muscles don't contract as easily (or at all), and we lose an impor-tant component of sexual participation and pleasure.

It stands to reason that if all these gruesome-sounding changes are the result of loss of estrogen, then estrogen replacement will re-verse them. It will. But estrogen has no effect on the libidinal aspects of our sexuality. That's where testosterone comes in. So let's bring this male hormone back onstage. How much do we lose, and how much do we miss it?

Our ovaries are not dead organs just because they stop producing estrogen. In about half of postmenopausal women, the ovaries continue to secrete substantial amounts of androgens, principally testosterone, for up to six years. If we compare the plasma levels of testosterone in women who have had their ovaries removed to those of naturally menopausal women, we find a significant difference. But significant is relative, and if we compare the amount of testosterone produced by menopausal women to that produced by younger women who are still menstruating, the levels in the menopausal women are lower. Because these women are not producing estrogen, even these lower levels of testosterone can take over because they are not bound up by SHBG. These may be the women who report a so-called menopausal zest—a renewed sense of well-being and sexual vigor after their periods have stopped. (Of course, the real reason could be that their kids are grown and they have the time, wherewithal and complete immunity from pregnancy that makes for great sex.)

Unfortunately, this group accounts for only half of naturally menopausal women. The other 50 percent of us lose it, and experience a rapid decline in ovarian testosterone production. The more overweight a woman is, the greater the likelihood she will suffer a decline in testosterone. Her abundant fat cells take the testosterone she is producing in her adrenal glands and convert it to estrogen. The good news is that the woman is less estrogen deficient. The bad news: She now has less testosterone, and what is left is being tied up and rendered inactive by increased levels of SHBG.

Now that we've reviewed all this scientifically collected and collated data, we have to conclude that from an ovarian point of view, many of us are testosterone-deprived, if not downright deficient. And we're feeling the effects.

NATURAL MENOPAUSE AND LOSS OF LIBIDO

Susan* is a 55-year-old film editor who has been in a good marriage for 24 years. Her periods stopped when she was 51, and she developed all of the symptoms of menopause—hot flashes, night sweats, insomnia, vaginal dryness and, as she put it, "mental fuzziness." She started hormone replacement therapy, taking Premarin (conjugated estrogen) each month from the first day to the 25th and Provera (progestin) from the 14th to the 25th. They worked, and Susan felt much better. Her sexual peppiness seemed undaunted, and she thought that she had successfully dealt with menopause.

But two years ago, Susan began to experience hot flashes and insomnia on her five days off Premarin, along with a gradual decrease in her sexual desire. Sex became less and less important, but she rationalized it's absence—she worked long days, was now in her mid-fifties and her husband was no longer that exciting. It took a lot of manual clitoral massage to get aroused, and orgasm was almost a non-event, so why bother? Susan's husband, who had always wanted to "bother" several times a week, now made fewer efforts to initiate sex. He was beginning to feel inadequate.

Initially, Susan didn't broach these issues with her doctor; after all, he was checking for more important medical problems like hypertension, diabetes, heart disease, osteoporosis and cancer. She was a good patient; she had every screening test a 55-year-old woman in charge of her health should have. What her doctor didn't ask she didn't tell. After all, how do you test or measure sex drive? When she finally mentioned that she didn't want or particularly enjoy sex, she was reassured that this was normal for someone her age. The "her age" did it, and she sought another opinion.

Susan's total testosterone levels were low and her free testosterone negligible. Her ovaries had finally quit responding to pituitary orders to make male hormone. Moreover, the estrogen she was taking was causing the testosterone she did produce to be bound up and rendered ineffectual. She felt reassured that there were hormonal reasons for her sexual apathy and wanted to see if male hormone replacement could help. I prescribed one-milligram methyltestosterone lozenges to be put under the tongue every day. I also suggested she take her Premarin on a daily basis so she would not develop hot flashes during the five non-estrogen days each month.

After eight weeks, Susan called me to report that there was a difference; at first it was subtle, but she definitely felt that some of her old pep and passion, as well as quality of orgasm, had returned. She has continued this therapy with improving results. After six months we checked her cholesteral profile; it was fine, unchanged from her previous exams.

Susan's menopause has not, after all, caused a sex-pause.

*Names and identifying details of all patients have been changed.

WHAT HAPPENS WHEN WE ARE TESTOSTERONE DEFICIENT?

The loss of testosterone during naturally occurring menopause is usually gradual. But much of what we know about the effects of testosterone deficiency comes from observing the symptoms that occur after sudden loss of testosterone due to surgical removal or chemical de-struction of the ovaries. In women who undergo a loss of ovaries, the drastic plunge of testosterone diminishes desire, intensity of sexual fantasies and sexual arousal. Tissues that are normally testosterone-sensitive, such as the nipples and clitoris, cease to evoke an erotic response and many women complain of "deadness" of the clitoris. Fantasy and masturbation no longer allow these women to reach or-gasm. Many complain of being unable to have orgasm no matter what the stimulation. And even if they achieve it, orgasm is shorter, more localized and less powerful. They no longer feel like having sex, they don't have the energy to do it and once they get started, the finish is disappointing.

Testosterone deficiency has a global effect: You don't just lose desire for your partner; you lose it for *any* partner, be it Tom Cruise or Sean Connery. There are also well-documented physical effects: thinning and loss of pubic hair; shrinking of genital tissues; dry, brit-tle skin and scalp hair; and loss of muscle tone. Headaches, depression and a diminished sense of well-being have been found to be signifi-cantly worse in women who have sudden loss of ovarian function due to surgery or chemotherapy and who are not treated with androgen replacement.

Having painted this bleak hormonal picture, I'll remind you that androgen deficiency is only one small corner of the sexual canvas. We need to realize that there are many other factors that define, promote or diminish our libido and sexuality, and we'll look at them in Part Two. But first let's consider the effect of low libido on the quality of our lives.

CHAPTER FOUR

"I'M NOT IN THE MOOD . . ."

⎯⎯⎯⎯⎯⎯⎯◡⎯⎯⎯⎯⎯⎯⎯

IT'S NOT "NICE" TO TALK OPENLY about our sex lives. Innuendo and jokes are exempt, of course (just look at any sitcom), but we feel that discretion is the better part of valor. So let's discreetly whisper about a secret we share: Most of us at some point in our lives feel that we are not reaching our biological sexual potential. We think we could do better, or should. We have acquired unrealistic expectations of what "better" is after being bombarded with images of waves crashing, bells ringing and birds singing. Let's get a grip here. We're all smart enough to realize that neither we nor our partners look like the actors on *Baywatch*, so why are we still convinced that our sexual responses and activities should be straight out of *Days of Our Lives?*

Fifty-six percent of women in the Janus study felt that they were not functioning at their sexual maximum. When asked to rate just how below-maximum they felt, more than half said they were operating at 50 percent or less of capacity. The incidence of persistently decreased libido in U.S. adults ranges from 11 to 48 percent, depending on which study you read, and a far greater percentage of people will have an isolated episode at some point in their life. In a 1997 study of 500 women ages 35 to 55 commissioned by *American Health for Women* magazine, 41 percent said they had experienced a temporary loss of interest in sex, 21 percent lacked desire for their partner and 10 percent had difficulty achieving orgasm. These numbers depend on whether a woman is expected to volunteer that she has a problem or is asked about it. Physicians who incorporate questions about sex in their medical history report that half their patients have low libido.

We're not meeting our expectations—no matter who defines them. But to further elucidate the extent of the problem and give it the medical credence it deserves, let's take a look at how the American Psychiatric Association, in its *Diagnostic and Statistical Manual of Mental Disorders*, classifies sexual dysfunction into four major categories:

(1) **Sexual desire disorders,** including hypoactive sexual desire (HSD) and sexual aversion disorder. HSD refers to a lack of responsiveness to sexual stimulation, a case of "persistently or recurrently deficient (or absent) sexual fantasies and desire for sexual activity." The prevalence of HSD in the overall population is estimated to be about 20 percent. Women are twice as likely as men to suffer from HSD, but that figure may reflect the fact that men may be less likely to acknowledge the problem and seek help. Sexual aversion disorder is a "persistent or recurrent extreme aversion to, and avoidance of, all (or almost all) genital sexual contact with a sexual partner." Obviously this makes any of the four stages of sexual response difficult if not impossible.

(2) **Sexual arousal disorders.** This term refers to a lack of responsiveness to sexual stimulation and is defined as "persistent or recurrent inability to attain, or to maintain until completion of sexual activity, an adequate lubrication-swelling response of sexual excitement." In women a sexual arousal disorder is similar to an erectile disorder in men.

(3) **Orgasmic disorders.** Generally regarded as one of the most common sexual dysfunctions in women, orgasmic disorders

are defined as "persistent or recurrent delay in, or absence of, orgasm following a normal sexual excitement phase." Prevalence rates of chronic inability to have an orgasm range from 5 to 10 percent of women, and it occurs more frequently in single than married or cohabitating women. According to *The Hite Report*, 70 percent of women have at some time in their lives been unable to have an orgasm. Of course, there is a wide variation in the frequency with which women climax, so in order to diagnose an orgasmic disorder, it is left up to the clinician to decide whether a woman's orgasmic capacity is less than what would be reasonable for her age, her sexual experience and the adequacy of stimulation. This is pretty arbitrary.

(4) **Sexual pain disorders,** including dyspareunia and vaginismus. Dyspareunia is defined as "recurrent or persistent genital pain associated with sexual intercourse" that is not caused by an underlying medical condition such as a vaginal infection. Vaginismus is "recurrent or persistent involuntary spasm of the musculature of the outer third of the vagina that interferes with sexual intercourse." In the National Health and Social Life survey, 15 percent of women of all ages reported pain during sex; in other studies of menopausal women who do not receive estrogen therapy, the number tops 40 percent.

To complicate matters, the American Psychiatric Association then groups these four classifications into psychological or medical, lifelong or acquired (developing after a period of normal sexual function) and generalized or situational (occurring only with a particular partner). All this looks very neat and tidy, but frequently we have to merge, combine and interface two or more of these sexual disorder diagnoses in order to arrive at an accurate description of what is really going on in an individual woman's life. A study of 588 male and female patients with an initial diagnosis of hypoactive sexual disorder, for example, demonstrated that 41 percent of females and 47 percent of males had at least one other sexual disorder diagnosis. And 18 percent of female patients had a diagnosis in all three categories of desire, arousal and orgasmic dysfunction.

It becomes extremely difficult for the physician to specify a diagnosis when the woman herself has difficulty determining what's missing. For example, she can't tell if she is orgasmic if she has problems becoming aroused in the first place. And if she is using a lubricant, she may not be able to determine if she lacks natural moisture. To make matters worse, the medical establishment doesn't always know what to do with each separate diagnosis, especially in women.

So there we have our definitions, our symptoms and some idea of the prevalence of these conditions. But how do they affect our lives and our relationships?

Sex is a way of reinforcing intimacy. When our sexuality is healthy, we often fail to notice how important it is. But when things aren't going well, bad sex may rule our relationship and indeed cause its demise. Sexual problems are a major reason for divorce, but the chicken-and-egg question is, "Which came first, a bad relationship, or bad sex?" Even in what the statisticians would call "normal" marriages, couples find that sex is disappointing or a downright failure 5 to 10 percent of the time. That doesn't mean that the marriage is doomed. But there is a point when it's appropriate to begin to worry. If you are having problems and they seem more frequent or persistent than in the past, don't ignore them. Here is a list of questions that may help you assess your sexual function and libido.

TAKING YOUR SEXUAL TEMPERATURE

1. Are you satisfied with your current level of function?
2. Do you or your partner have any concerns about how often you engage in sex?
3. Do you have any trouble achieving orgasm? How frequently does that occur?
4. Does your partner have any problems achieving or maintaining erections?
5. Are you and your partner able to talk comfortably about your sexual relationship?

If the answers to the above give a clear indication that your libido and sexual relationship are in jeopardy, consider going over this next set of questions with your physician.

A SEXUAL HEALTH CHECKLIST

1. How would you rate your current sexual function on a scale of 1 to 10, with 1 being nonfunctional and 10 being superb?
2. When did you first notice a decrease in your libido?
3. Has the frequency of sex with your partner changed? Does your partner want to have sex more or less frequently than you?
4. When you do have sex with your partner, do you enjoy it? Are you able to reach orgasm?
5. Can you achieve orgasm through masturbation and fantasy?
6. Are you able to feel aroused when you see an erotic movie, read a sexy book or look at pictures of gorgeous men? Or does nothing strike your interest?
7. Have you experienced orgasms in the past?
8. Do you feel it's taking you longer and there is more work involved to reach orgasm than in the past?
9. Do you lack lubrication? Does sex hurt?

10. How many children have you had? How young are they, and are you currently breast-feeding?

11. What are you using for contraception?

12. Are your periods still regular? Do you have increasing PMS or are you experiencing hot flashes?

13. Do you have any medical problems?

14. Have you noticed a sudden change in your weight? Are you happy with your weight?

15. Do you think of yourself as an attractive sex partner?

16. Are you exercising? How much?

17. How much alcohol do you drink?

18. Do you smoke?

19. Have you or your partner had any sexually transmitted diseases? Do the symptoms tend to recur?

20. Are you currently taking any medications?

21. Does your partner have any medical or erection problems?

22. How would you define your marriage/relationship with your partner? Has it changed over the last few years?

23. Do you think your partner is monogamous?

24. How would you describe your current stress level?

25. Is life bleak, or just sex?

26. Do you recall any instances of fondling or sexual abuse as a youngster or has sex ever been forced on you?

27. When you were growing up, were you told that good girls did not have sex until they became married?

These questions will help you and your doctor to delineate the causes of your sexual troubles and go on to the next step, therapy—so that "I'm not in the mood . . ." is not a permanent condition.

DIMINISHED LIBIDO AND LOW TESTOSTERONE—BUT WE DON'T KNOW WHY

Dina is a 40-year-old married homemaker. She has had two children and delivered her last (all 10 pounds of him) ten years ago. Although she had vaginal lacerations with the delivery, she doesn't feel that the area is overstretched and does not have vaginal pain. Since this last delivery, she has had diminished sex drive and over the past few months, she hasn't been able to get aroused at all. Dina does everything she can to avoid having intercourse, and this has caused marital difficulties. About a year ago, she started taking Paxil for severe PMS. She doesn't think the antidepressant worsened her sex drive; as she puts it, "Zero minus zero still equals zero." Her menstrual cycles have become very light and, of late, she has started to have night sweats.

On examination, I felt that Dina was right—there did not seem to be any vaginal scarring or abnormal prolapse from her last delivery. Her uterus was normal in size and I felt no ovarian masses. From a gynecologic standpoint, she was fine. Her blood count and thyroid were in the normal range; she had normal levels of FSH, estrogen and DHEAS, but her free testosterone was low at 0.7 picograms per milliliter (normal range is 0.8 to 3.2). There is no way to know if Dina's current low testosterone explains her diminished libido for the past 10 years, but feeling we had nothing to lose, I prescribed testosterone propionate 2-percent ointment. I have also referred her to our sexual therapist, who may be able to delve into the more complex issues of her body image and sexual feelings subsequent to her delivery. The therapist will work with Dina on maximizing fantasy and give her suggestions on ways to increase arousal. If all of this is not enough, Dina may have to go off the Paxil, which has been shown to dull libido, and try other therapies for PMS such as herbs, vitamins and exercise. Dina is willing; she has become an expert on intercourse avoidance, and it's a skill she wants to lose.

PART TWO

THE
SEVEN SEXUAL
SABOTEURS

CHAPTER FIVE

PSYCHOLOGICAL ISSUES

It should be clear that we can't blame hormones for all our sexual woes any more than we can blame PMS for every bad mood or menopause for any complaint that occurs after the age of 50. Before we begin a massive rush to test our testosterone levels or badger our physician to prescribe this hormone, we have to consider the other major factors in our life that can undermine our sexual pleasure and sexual health. A chief suspect: psychological concerns.

Sexuality has occupied a central role in the field of psychology ever since the father of psychoanalysis, Sigmund Freud, hypothesized that our sexual instincts were the driving force in our personality. If these forces went awry, he theorized, our psyches would end up doing the same. Current thinking reverses the cause and effect: Psychological neuroses and psychoses influence our sexuality. Anxiety, guilt and extreme self-consciousness, for example, negatively affect our sexual expression, whereas sociability, confidence, rashness, exhibitionism and dominance positively facilitate it (well, maybe the last three aren't so positive).

DEPRESSION

The problem: Twenty percent of women develop depression at some point in their lifetime, and we outdepress men by a factor of two to one. This incidence may increase in the perimenopause, at which point we reach a ratio of three or four to one! Depression is associated with tearfulness, excessive worry and anxiety, food cravings, increased appetite, appetite changes, decreased energy, poor sleep and emotional detachment. Any of these will put us "out of the mood."

We now know that depression is associated with changes in the brain chemicals dopamine and serotonin, as well as in the adrenal hormone cortisol. Shifts in the latter can diminish central production of FSH and LH and secretion of testosterone, estrogen and progesterone, so we may ultimately get a central hormonal depression and depressed desire.

Approach to therapy: We have to treat our depression before we can treat our sexual problem. Psychotherapy alone will help 45 to 60 percent of women with mild to moderate depression, and some degree of psychotherapy is always indicated if only to ascertain who among us will benefit from medication. Unfortunately, in these days of HMOs, PPOs and harried primary care providers, throwing pills at us is a lot easier and cheaper than talking about the problem and referring us for counseling. (The tossed-about drugs can have their own negative impact on our sexual desire and function, but more on that in Chapter 7.) A combination of medication and psychotherapy is warranted if we get an inadequate response from one or the other, and this should benefit 50 to 60 percent of women with severe or recurrent depression. In the case of perimenopausal or menopausal women, whose depressed mood may be exacerbated by fluctuating or decreasing estrogen levels, the medication should include estrogen.

Indeed, it has been found that estrogen boosts the response to psychotropic drugs in menopausal women.

STRESS AND ANXIETY

The problem: Sudden, severe stress (the kind that triggers the body's fight-or-flight response) and chronic stress (the cumulative effect of day-to-day problems) can each have long-term consequences for our bodies, psyches and libidos. The physical toll of stress is enormous and includes fatigue, lack of energy, irritability and hostility, none of which makes us feel sexy. From a chemical point of view, acute stress causes a spike in our stress hormone levels, and when this happens repeatedly, levels of these hormones never completely return to normal. Over time, this can inhibit ovarian activity and production of sex hormones, including testosterone. It can also directly affect our brain's centers for sexual behavior.

In groups of monkeys, the most subordinate males have the lowest levels of testosterone, while subordinate females become desensitized to pituitary hormones and don't ovulate properly. What about groups of humans? There is some good evidence that extreme physical or psychological stress can lower testosterone; however, the research that demonstrated this effect was done mostly in men. It appears that whenever physical or psychological stress was quantified it had to do with combat, military academies or athletic training. Nobody bothered to quantify childbirth or child rearing.

Here is what we do know about women's sexual response to stress: Women with hypoactive sexual desire report significantly higher levels of stress than men, and those of us caught between the dual demands of work and family life may be especially at risk. Researchers have found that women employed in professional positions are more likely to experience this problem than women in nonprofessional positions or those who are not employed.

Sex-related difficulties can themselves be stressors, and infertility is one of the three biggest culprits (infidelity and sexual dysfunction are the other two). Not only can hormones used to stimulate ovulation in infertile women decrease libido, but the pressure to have sex on schedule for purposes of procreation rather than pleasure may worsen the situation. Half of couples undergoing in-vitro fertilization report that infertility is the most upsetting experience of their lives.

Whatever the cause of the stress, its negative effect on our sexuality becomes a self-perpetuating cycle. When we fail to become aroused or achieve orgasm, we become anxious about future encounters. Our lowered expectations may come true: We fail yet again to perform or respond adequately, and our libido goes into a tailspin.

Approach to therapy: I don't have any easy answers. (As a matter of fact, the pressure to complete this book on time has left me searching for solutions myself.) Dealing with major life stresses such as birth, death, marriage, divorce, financial hardship, a new job or children moving out (or worse yet, moving back in) depletes us emotionally and requires enormous adjustments. It's unfair to expect that sex will continue as usual. Our first priority is to make sure we regain our mental and physical health.

Life-changing events are not the only ones that can take a toll. The cumulative effect of everyday hassles can be just as damaging. No matter what type of stress we're dealing with, we must make time to cultivate the intimacy and affection that will help us cope with life and regain our sexuality. Studies of the effects of stress on our bodies have shown that exercise, proper diet, relaxation techniques, psychotherapy and even medication can prevent long-term damage. (Unfortunately, some of those stress-easing drugs can have sex-impairing effects of their own.)

SEXUAL ABUSE

The problem: Up to 23 percent of women have suffered some form of sexual abuse. Subsequently they are more likely than other women to lack interest or pleasure in sex, have pain during intercourse or fail to achieve orgasm. Furthermore these women are at increased risk for depression, chronic anxiety, substance abuse and low self-esteem, all of which can also result in sexual dysfunction. The trauma of childhood sexual abuse is often equated with the more medically examined combat-related post-traumatic stress disorder (PTSD). In PTSD, the pathway that links the brain, pituitary and adrenal glands functions abnormally and, as a result, the body loses some of its natural ability to control the output of stress hormones. This failure to react leads to hormonal apathy and finally behavioral and sexual apathy.

For some survivors, any sexual contact can cause flashbacks— vivid images or memories of the assault. This shuts off all desire and leads to avoidance of physical intimacy. Between 63 and 85 percent of women who have experienced childhood sexual abuse report some sexual difficulties in adulthood, and a recent study found that those whose abuse had involved penetration or physical force had the most severe problems.

Approach to therapy: Women with PTSD-related sexual problems have great difficulty allowing the barriers they have built against sexual feelings to be torn down. They tend to resist any sexual therapy until they have worked on uncovering the initial damaging experience and exploring its effect on their psychological and sexual development in intensive therapy. Only after this detoxification process can sexual problems be confronted.

THE FATIGUE FACTOR

Miriam is 26 years old, married and studying to be a rabbi. She attends classes six to eight hours a day, diligently does her homework, is in charge of all the shopping and cooking (her husband feels he's excused because he's getting a Ph.D.) and is lucky if she gets six hours of sleep a night. She has a history of recurrent tonsillitis and frequently needs to take antibiotics. She also takes Demulin birth control pills. She came to see me complaining of recurrent yeast infections, vaginal dryness and general fatigue, and added that she had a very low libido for the past few years.

When I examined her, Miriam had just finished a course of the antibiotic Zithromax, and when I examined her I found reddening and puffiness around the labia and a white discharge which, on microscopy, showed yeast. Other than that, her cervix, uterus and ovaries were normal. A complete blood count showed no anemia, although her iron levels were low, and her thyroid function was normal. Her free testosterone level was in the low normal range. After treating Miriam's yeast infection, I suggested she switch her monophasic birth control pill, Demulen, to a tricyclic pill, OrthoTri-Cyclen. Since birth control pills can increase propensity for yeast infections, I told her if these infections recur (and she is not taking antibiotics, which can also lead to yeast infections), she might need to go off the Pill entirely. Although oral contraceptives can diminish libido, I think the main culprit is Miriam's lifestyle, lack of sleep and stress. I suggested she take vitamins pills with iron, try to get some exercise and plan to spend some quality hours with her husband on the weekends. The dual libido insults of stress and fatigue in Miriam's life won't radically change until she finishes school (and then, of course, there is her future work as a rabbi and starting a family—oy vey, it will never be easy!). She will see me in six months and report whether she feels any better on her new birth control pills.

BODY IMAGE ISSUES

EATING DISORDERS

The problem: Anorexia, bulimia and inappropriate dieting are depressingly common in women. They tend to begin in adolescence but may continue throughout life. Two percent of adolescent girls are anorexic, at least 8 percent are bulimic and, at any given time, at least 50 percent are dieting. Weight loss associated with eating disorders affects hormone levels throughout the body. A 10 percent loss of ideal body weight can cause women to stop ovulating and menstruating and produce less estrogen and testosterone. To compound this hormonal insult, the adrenal glands may also shut down—and there goes our last resource for testosterone. The result is vaginal atrophy and diminished arousal.

Should we care if 14- to 18-year-olds (the peak age group for anorexia) have diminished libido? Yes, because the associated poor body image and lack of self-worth set the sexual tone for the future. Furthermore, it can take years for a woman who gains back weight to reestablish regular menstrual cycles and hormone levels. Many of these women may seem healthy according to the scale, but never completely stabilize their eating habits, body image or hormone levels.

Approach to therapy: The first step is to treat the problem eating pattern, often with psychotherapy and antidepressants. It is also paramount for both present and future health (including sexual health) that we correct hormonal deficiencies and reestablish regular cycles. This will prevent vaginal dryness and reduce the risk of osteoporosis and heart disease. These estrogen-deficient young women should be treated with low-dose birth control pills or hormone replacement therapy. We don't yet know whether testosterone should be added to the mix.

OBESITY

The problem: Thirty-seven percent of American women are clinically obese. We know what this does to our health, but how does it affect our sexual health? In the *American Health for Women* survey, 23 percent of women said they felt too fat for sex. Other studies have shown that women who rate themselves negatively on something called a "sexual self schema scale," which includes questions about body image and weight, see themselves as less romantic, passionate and open to sexual experience than do women with a positive self-rating. Obese women describe themselves as self-conscious and embarrassed and may feel that their self-image is strongly defined by others. In our society, obesity may be a greater "sin" than sex.

Since most of us tend to put on weight in midlife, we're dealt a sexual double-whammy: Just as we're confronting the fact that we no longer meet our culture's beauty ideal, we are also coping with diminished production of testosterone. But the hormonal picture gets even more complex. On one hand, estrogen is produced in fat cells, so the fatter we are the more estrogen we have. This in turn decreases our percentage of unbound, active testosterone, which could diminish our libido. On the other hand, fat also causes us to become insulin-resistant: Levels of insulin rise until we exhaust our ability to produce this hormone (hence the connection between obesity and diabetes). High levels of insulin increase male hormone production. How do these average out? Do women who are about to develop diabetes have a stronger libido? No one knows, but I suspect that weight gain's damage to our self-image overpowers any possible boost in libido that would result from an increase in our male hormone.

Approach to therapy: I could lecture you on weight loss, and I certainly don't want to diminish its importance to your health, but this is not a diet book. My advice is to set realistic goals, such as a 10-percent weight loss, and to concentrate on being fit, eating properly and staying healthy. But even as we are doing this it is also necessary to reevaluate how we feel about our bodies. Our physical ability to become aroused, achieve sexual satisfaction and reciprocate is there no matter what our weight. We have to stop focusing on what society tells us is beautiful and concentrate instead on what we find beautiful and pleasurable about ourselves. There are myriad body image workshops, books and exercises that can help you do this (see Resources and Recommended Readings); if self-help tactics don't work, consult a therapist.

CHAPTER SIX

COUPLE TROUBLE

EMOTIONAL ISSUES AND REJECTION by a partner have been blamed by 40 percent of women and 43 percent of men for the breakup of their marriage. Divorce may be the end result, but sexual problems often precede it. Thirty-five percent of divorced women state that sex became worse after marriage, and I can't help but suspect that lack of sexual gratification played some part in the breakup. That doesn't mean that all women who remain married are sexually satisfied. Indeed, 11 percent of them state that gratification went downhill after the wedding. Let's look at some of the couple problems that can have sexual repercussions.

RELATIONSHIP DIFFICULTIES

The problem: We often ignore relationship problems in our twenties and thirties, while we're raising our children, building our career and paying our mortgage. But once the children have left the home and we no longer have to struggle to pay for it (although we may still be struggling to pay for their education), our marital troubles can become magnified, sometimes to the point where we question the need for a relationship. There are those of us who are workaholics or who feel our obligations overwhelm our time and priorities. We forget the romantic and sexual spark that brought us together with our mate in the first place. Our relationship becomes a business partnership, where we share housekeeping, financial and social obligations, but not intimacy. We are too exhausted from our other pursuits to even think about sex. We get out of the habit and subsequently lose desire.

Approach to therapy: Make a weekly date for sex (calendar permitting, you can of course make it more frequent) and set aside a special time to spend together outside the bedroom. On the appointed day, make this time one of your three top priorities; otherwise you won't get to it. If you're too exhausted at the end of a busy day to have sex, switch your schedule and plan to have intercourse in the morning before your energies are depleted by more mundane events. (If your problems are persistent, see Chapter 14 for more suggestions.) Even in the "best" of marriages, intimacy and passion are fleeting and fragile and cannot be taken for granted.

POWER ISSUES

The problem: If we don't feel respected and important, it's natural to respond with anger and resentment. And if that anger is left unresolved, it can gradually dampen desire and arousal, and this can become chronic. Studies have shown that women react to anger with greater loss of libido than men. After all, if we don't feel loved outside the bedroom, why should we want to make love in it? (This seems to be less of a problem for men.) This type of libido deficiency is very specific: We're only mad at one male, so it does not prevent our fantasizing about someone else (or even acting on these fantasies). Sometimes we even use this loss of desire—often unconsciously—to get back at our partner. When we say we don't want sex, our partner is left feeling undesirable and wounded. That may even the score, but we're both left wanting.

Power struggles aren't always about anger; they can be due to the natural variations in libido between two people. For some of us, making love once a week is great, while for others, five times is the goal.

The one wanting more sex may be the one with the problem. He (or sometimes she) might be using sex as a sort of physical Xanax, to relax him when he's anxious, as a pick-me-up when he's bored or as a way to make sure he's getting attention from his partner. When differing levels of sexual interest occur, especially when they weren't present in the past, they may be a sign of a serious relationship problem.

The ultimate inequity, of course, is when one partner has an extramarital affair. At first, the discovery of the infidelity may stimulate sexual behavior, but the end result is likely to be lack of trust, followed by low libido—and possibly a call to 1 (800) DIVORCE.

Approach to therapy: It's important to open a line of communication between the partners so that anger can be expressed in places other than the bedroom. (For suggestions on ways to get started talking to one another, see Chapter 14.) When it comes to different levels of desire, negotiation (and ensuing adjustment to more realistic expectations) is in order. As for infidelity, get thee to a marriage counselor (it's up to you to decide if a divorce attorney is more appropriate) and see your gynecologist to get tested for sexually transmitted diseases. Until you're sure that your partner has returned to monogamy, condoms are in order.

LACK OF CHEMISTRY

The problem: The song "Love Potion #9" may make us sing and dance, but it's not what we play when we march down the aisle. When it comes to choosing a mate, we often look for qualities such as kindness, generosity, stability and financial success not to mention shared ethnicity, religious background and interests. But if there is no chemical attraction in the beginning and sex was never good, it

LACK OF CHEMICAL ATTRACTION

Cindy is 34 years old. She and her husband have been married for six years and have had sex eight times. Prior to the relationship, they both had active, pleasurable sex lives. Cindy's last boyfriend left her with a recurrent memento of the relationship—herpes. She met her husband three years before they got married, and they both decided that they would not have sex until the wedding; instead, they would work on common pursuits and bonds.

Cindy and her husband go hiking together; they like the same music, love to cook, travel together, and get along "just fine." But when it comes to sex, she experiences zero attraction. In her own words, she feels, "my husband is more like my brother." She does fantasize and feels aroused when she sees an erotic movie or a sexy man. She can achieve orgasm with masturbation.

It's clear that Cindy shows no signs of androgen deficiency. She manifests chronic "husband excitement deficiency." Even after we discussed this, she wanted clinical corroboration. After all, there must be a hormone she can take to fix this sexual disinterest—"He's such a great guy," she says. So, I tested her free testosterone level (normal), her thyroid function (normal) and her DHEAS (also normal). Needless to say, her physical gynecological exam was fine. I referred Cindy and her husband to a sex therapist; Cindy was not sure they would go.

will become extremely difficult to initiate interest down the line. Lack of intimacy becomes a source of constant tension and stress, and can ultimately doom a relationship that, on paper and to the outside world, looks great. (How many times have you said to yourself, "They were such a great couple . . . why did they break up?")

Approach to therapy: Sexual attraction is so fundamental that in this case the best thing to do may be to acknowledge that the problem exists and decide whether you can live with it. You might want to try working with a sex therapist, but the results for this particular problem tend to be discouraging.

CHAPTER SEVEN

MEDICATIONS

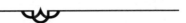

THE EXTENT TO WHICH DRUGS can have an effect on our sexual behavior and libido has been underappreciated for several reasons. Most of the studies that link medications with sexual dysfunction have been carried out on men, whose dysfunction is plain to see. Although they are rarely cited as a medical side effect and may not have the same magnitude, engorgement and arousal problems in women are akin to erectile difficulties in men. After all, increased blood flow and swelling of the clitoris, vulva and vagina is similar to that of the penis, and what affects one most likely affects the other. So from here on in (with the exception of Chapter 11), when I talk about erectile dysfunction, I am speaking chiefly of arousal difficulties in women.

The next problem regarding drugs and sex lies in the reporting of medication side effects: During clinical trials, patients are rarely asked if they noticed any sexual difficulties after they began taking the drug or placebo. Although scientifically less acceptable, case reports by sensitive clinicians who inquire about sexual behavior may tell us more than controlled studies that rely on patients' self-evaluation.

Doctors and pharmacologists also don't understand the mechanism through which many drugs might influence sexual function because we don't fully understand the physiology of sex in the first place. Many drugs have both a direct effect on our brain and central nervous system and a local effect on our genitalia, and on occasion the drug's action on one may contradict its effect on the other. For example, an antidepressant might boost our mood and make us more likely to want sex, yet if it increases serotonin levels in the brain we wind up with lowered libido. Birth control pills might correct certain hormonal imbalances but may also diminish testosterone levels and libido. On a more local basis, some women find birth control pills increase vaginal lubrication while others find the opposite to be true, especially if they develop more yeast infections and pain with intercourse. Having posed this paradox, let's consider the paltry information that has been gathered when it comes to women, medications and libido. Let's also look at some of the drugs that have been shown to cause impotence in men. Until more is known, we have to assume that they effect our sexual response as well.

BIRTH CONTROL PILLS AND OTHER HORMONES

The problem: Fifteen million American women are currently taking oral contraceptives, and the implications of any effect on libido are enormous. Yet the studies that exist of the Pill–libido link are on very small numbers of women. Who is going to pay for them? Not the pharmaceutical companies! Here is what we do know: A 1974 British study found that women using oral contraceptives were four times more likely to complain of sexual difficulties than women using other birth control methods. But these women were on much higher-dose pills than we currently use, and because they were seeing physicians for regular follow-up visits they were more likely than women who didn't get Pill checkups to report sexual problems.

Because the Pill suppresses ovarian activity, it potentially lowers production of male hormone. This effect is compounded by the estrogen in the Pill, which increases SHBG and will further lower free testosterone. Yet a small study comparing two groups of 20 women on the Pill, one with sexual difficulties and one without, showed no difference between their androgen levels. Moreover, giving the women with sexual difficulties male hormones didn't help. Another intriguing piece of information: During the Pill-free week of their cycle, many of the women reported a surge in sexual interest, and it was found that their testosterone levels were higher during this time.

It's possible that if the Pill diminishes libido, it goes unreported because women sense the problem quickly and stop taking the drug after only a few months, before anyone—including researchers—has had a chance to talk to them. The Pill might also undermine libido (and unfortunately, we're still hypothesizing here) through its progestin. Although the progestin-only mini-pill and the progestin-containing Norplant implant have not been implicated in depressed desire, a recent study of Depo-Provera, a long-lasting injectable progestin, found that 8 percent of users experienced this side effect. Equating one pill with another may be a libidinal injustice. Some pills contain progestins that are more androgenic than others, and thus might be better for sex (the down side is that they can cause more mood swings and acne). Triphasic pills, which give three different levels of progestin at different points in the cycle, may cause less suppression of normal androgen fluctuation than monophasic pills, which deliver a steady dose. Indeed, a 1996 study by San Francisco State University showed that triphasic users experienced fewer libido changes than monophasic users.

Approach to therapy: If you feel less lusty since you started taking a monophasic birth control pill (Ortho-Novum, Ovral, Lo-Ovral, Demulen, Levlen, Ovcon, Desogen, Ortho-Cept, Nordette, Alesse, Mircette, Loestrin or Norinyl), ask your doctor about changing to one that's triphasic (Ortho Tri-Cyclen, Ortho-Novum 7-7-7, Triphasyl, Tri-Levlen or Tri-Norinyl). If you are taking a pill with a low androgenic progestin or low androgenic activity (Desogen, Ortho-Cept,

OrthoCyclen, Demulen/35, Ovcon 35 or Mircette), you might switch to one with higher male hormone activity, such as Lo-Ovral, Nordette, Levlen or Ortho-Novum 35. And if these new combinations and permutations don't help, stop the Pill, use another method of birth control and see if it makes a difference.

HORMONE REPLACEMENT THERAPY

The problem: We have already dealt with the effect of estrogen replacement on menopausal women: It decreases vaginal dryness and atrophy and helps prevent discomfort with intercourse. But women who take estrogen will have lower free testosterone levels as SHBG rises and binds up whatever testosterone they are producing. So even though estrogen is good for genital health, it may upset the delicate balance of total and free testosterone, and in women who are perilously close to having too little may cause libidinous changes.

"Designer estrogens," or selective estrogen receptor modulators (SERMs), have recently been featured in news reports because of their potential to decrease onset or prevent recurrence of breast cancer. Like estrogen, tamoxifen and raloxifene (Evista) may interfere with the bioavailability of testosterone. Many women complain that tamoxifen increases vaginal discharge. Neither SERM will prevent menopause-related vaginal dryness and atrophy.

Progestins are used in combination with estrogen for women who still have a uterus. The bad news is that by the age of menopause, one-third of us have already had a hysterectomy. The good news is that we then don't have to worry about progestins. As usual (I'm getting tired of saying this), we have no good data correlating progestins with changes in desire. We do know, however, that synthetic medroxyprogesterone acetate (MPA, Provera or Cycrin) has been associated with increased PMS-like complaints. Bloating, depression and headaches are not sex promoters. The natural progesterones

(Prometrium or those made by compounding pharmacies) may eliminate these side effects, but they can cause drowsiness.

Approach to therapy: If we take hormone replacement therapy (HRT), we may be enhancing loss of active testosterone that occurs in this transition. However, we have some very profound health reasons to use it. In the short term, estrogen can control hot flashes, vaginal dryness, sleep disturbances, mood changes, skin changes and memory lapses and give us a general sense of well-being (wow!). And long term, it will help protect us from cardiovascular disease, osteoporosis, Alzheimer's disease and perhaps colon cancer. So it doesn't make sense to stop solely because of a diminished libido. This is where testosterone supplementation should be considered (see Chapter 12).

ANTIHORMONES (GnRH ANALOGS AND DANAZOL)

The problem: The GnRH analogs Lupron and Synarel are used to control endometriosis, uterine fibroids, heavy bleeding and severe PMS. They pretend to be the gonadotropic releasing hormone (GnRH) that stimulates pituitary production of FSH and LH. The analogs sit on GnRH receptors and block the access of the real thing, so the brain no longer signals the ovaries to produce hormones—and we develop chemical menopause. Because of ovarian shutdown, we develop the obvious side effects due to loss of estrogen; we can also expect some loss of libido. In real life this doesn't always occur, because the drug is used in younger women whose adrenals are still producing what may be adequate amounts of testosterone. Another plus: These drugs are usually prescribed for short periods of time (up to six months), so any effects should be temporary. Like GnRH analogs, Danazol, which is also used to treat endometriosis, suppresses signals from the pituitary to the ovary. It has a weak male hormone–like activity and has been shown to both increase and decrease libido.

Approach to therapy: Estrogen and progesterone replacement therapy is currently being prescribed for many women taking GnRH analogs, especially if they are being treated for more than a few months. It stands to reason that if necessary, testosterone could be included in this "add back" regime. Because the menopausal side effects of Danazol are not as strong as those of the GnRH analogs, hormone replacement is not given.

ANTIDEPRESSANTS

The problem: The chief culprits seem to be the selective serotonin reuptake inhibitors (SSRIs), which increase serotonin levels in the brain. We know that low serotonin is associated with depression and that depression curtails libido. So if we eliminate the depression, shouldn't we lift our libido? Raising the levels of this neurochemical may make us feel happier, more relaxed and less anxious, but unfortunately it has the opposite effect on sexual desire. The link between serotonin and sex is poorly understood, but it is possible that serotonin diminishes dopamine, one of the brain's pleasure chemicals. There is also evidence that serotonin decreases testosterone levels. Low levels of serotonin cause female rats to take more initiative, mount other female rats and smaller males and in general act more like males. So when we raise our serotonin levels (if we compare ourselves with female rodents) we may lose sexual aggression.

At least 58 percent of SSRI users (women and men) report sexual dysfunction when specifically asked about it by researchers. Initially the reports zeroed in on Prozac, but as more SSRIs have been developed, we've seen a libido effect from others, including Zoloft, Luvox and Paxil.

Other commonly prescribed non-SSRI antidepressants, such as tricyclics and monoamine oxidase (MAO) inhibitors, have also been reported to cause decreased libido. These include amitriptyline, desipramine, doxepin, imipramine, nortriptyline, phenelzine and protriptyline. But it is often difficult to pinpoint the cause of the problem, because the underlying condition of depression has such a dampening effect on sex.

Approach to therapy: Sometimes it is sufficient simply to lower the dose to the point where we feel better sexually without sacrificing any of the drug's psychological benefits. Another option is to take a "drug holiday," stopping the medication on weekends or before a romantic getaway (this should be done only after consultation with your physician). It may also be helpful to take the medication after, rather than before, lovemaking. If these methods fail, the libido issue might be resolved by switching medications. An antidepressant that appears to have little or no antisexual side effects is Wellbutrin. In one study, 80 percent of patients who experienced lack of orgasm while taking Prozac had a return of normal function when switched to Wellbutrin. In some cases, doctors are now giving Wellbutrin together with an SSRI as a kind of "cocktail" to benefit both depression and libido. An older SSRI, Desyrel, may actually increase libido in depressed individuals, but it has a rare side effect: prolonged, uncomfortable swelling of blood vessels in the clitoris or penis.

If substitution or addition of Wellbutrin is not an option or doesn't help, it is possible to add low doses of yohimbine, a plant-derived substance that has been shown to block the antilibido and erectile effects of SSRIs (see Chapter 13). Or a physician can prescribe amantadine (sold under the brand name Symmetrel), a medication known by many of us for its flu-fighting capabilities and also used in the treatment of Parkinson's disease. Taken five to six hours before intercourse, amantadine can increase the brain's level of dopamine, promoting libido. Cyproheptadine (marketed as Perioactin), a prescription antihistamine, is also an antiserotonin (i.e., it will lower serotonin levels) and may help. It should be taken a few hours before sex or as a daily dose. Unfortunately, it too has side effects: Cyproheptadine can cause sleepiness and may even reverse the effects of antidepressants. Urecholine, a medication given to help the bladder contract, has been reported to reverse anorgasmia from tricyclic antidepressants if taken one to two hours prior to sex.

ANTIPSYCHOTICS

The problem: Most of us don't feel we need antipsychotic drugs, but they should be included in any list of drugs that decrease libido and/or prevent orgasm and cause erectile dysfunction. Some of these medications may block dopamine activity in the brain; they can also increase prolactin levels, which in turn lowers testosterone and libido. Others could have a more local effect. The list of tranquilizers that affect sexual function is long, and includes thioridazine, chlorpromazine, chlorprothixine, mesoridazine, perphenazine and trifluoperazine.

Approach to therapy: Consult a psychiatrist or a psychopharmacologist (a psychiatrist who specializes in the intricate chemistry of psychiatric medications) for advice on drugs that can be substituted. For example, thorazine may interfere with orgasm more frequently than other antipsychotic drugs.

TRANQUILIZERS

The problem: All tranquilizers probably are capable of disrupting sexual function. There have been reports of decreased libido, erectile problems and lack of orgasm associated with most of them. This is probably due to a combination of central nervous system effects like sedation, local effects on the genitals and excessive muscle relaxation. Commonly used tranquilizers include chlordiazepoxide, lorazepam and alprazolam. Clonazepam, marketed under the name Klonopin, is a benzodiazepine that is used as an antidepressant as well as for seizure and panic disorders. In one study it was found to be associated with sexual side effects in over 90 percent of patients.

Approach to therapy: As with antidepressants, consider lowering the dose or switching to another medication. BuSpar may have less severe antisexual effects than some of the other drugs.

MOOD STABILIZERS

The problem: Lithium is suspect when it comes to interfering with libido and erection, but no link has been demonstrated between lithium levels and sexual function. A recent study showed that patients who took lithium plus Valium had high rates of sexual dysfunction, while those given lithium alone had fewer difficulties. The sexual side effects of anticonvulsant mood stabilizers such as Depakote (valproic acid, used to treat epilepsy and prevent migraine) and Tegretol have been poorly studied. We do know, however, that Tegretol lowers free testosterone levels and we suspect that this may result in diminished libido.

Approach to therapy: Since Depakote doesn't seem to alter metabolism of our sex hormones, it may be the preferred drug if sexual dysfunction becomes an issue.

BLOOD-PRESSURE-LOWERING MEDICATIONS

The problem: Drugs that lower blood pressure probably interfere with our sexual function more often than any other type of medication, because so many of us are on them. These drugs affect the central nervous system and levels of important neurotransmitters such as dopamine; they may also impair impulses to the genitalia and prevent rapid blood flow to the area during arousal. Even diuretics, which are frequently used to treat mild hypertension (and bloating) in women, may have an anti-erectile effect in anywhere from 3 to 36 percent of users.

One mild antihypertensive and diuretic, spironolactone, is known to block the action of testosterone and is therefore used to treat acne and excessive hair growth (hirsutism) in women. It too is associated with libido and erection disturbances, probably because of its anti-male-hormone effects. Beta-blocking drugs (brand names include Inderal, Lopressor and Tenormin), used both to lower blood pressure and treat heart disease, may cause erectile failure. Another commonly used cardiac medicine, digoxin, may cause diminished libido and arousal. Blood-pressure-lowering medications that are potentially libido lowering include clonidine, methyldopa, guanethedine and reserpine.

Approach to therapy: I am not suggesting you risk a heart attack or stroke in order to preserve your sex drive. On the other hand, exercise, proper diet, weight loss and a limited sodium intake will help prevent the former and certainly won't hurt the latter. If your libido or arousal problems began at the same time you started any of these medications, talk to your physician about trying alternative drugs to see if you can find one that has fewer sexual side effects.

OTHER MEDICINES

Here is a depressingly long "A" list of medications that many of us take at one time or another. These drugs have all been shown to be capable of causing loss of libido, erectile dysfunction, inhibition of orgasm or diminished genital sensation, so it is paramount that we become drug detectives and try to pinpoint any onset of sexual disturbance to the use of these medications. We may enter the pharmacy with our sexuality intact, but we risk leaving it with a product that may be harmful to our sexual health.

- **Antacids:** Cimetidine (Tagamet), famotidine (Pepcid), ranitidine (Zantac), nizatidine (Axid), omeprazole (Prilosec)
- **Anti-alcohol:** Disulfuram, given to treat alcoholism
- **Antibiotics:** Broad-spectrum antibiotics given for upper-respiratory tract, gastrointestinal and bladder infections can change our natural vaginal flora, resulting in irritation and discomfort with intercourse.
- **Anticholesterol:** Gemfibrozil (Lopid)
- **Anti-epileptic:** Phenytoin (Dilantin)
- **Antifungal:** Ketoconazole (Nizoral)
- **Antihistamines:** Over-the-counter cold and allergy remedies can dry us up, both in our upper airways and lower vagina, and are at fault for decreased lubrication. Remember they also can cause drowsiness.
- **Anti-inflammatories:** Naproxen (Anaprox, Naprosyn)

RECREATIONAL DRUGS

The problem: Current recommendations for medical use of marijuana do not include treatment of sexual dysfunction! It would be dishonest to deny that this drug may produce a temporary increase in libido and sexual prowess. However, chronic use of marijuana or any legal (narcotics, barbiturates) or illegal (cocaine, heroin, LSD) substance of abuse can lead to sexual impairment.

As for that other recreational drug, alcohol, which many of us have used to lessen inhibition: All it will do is cause us to feel tired and depressed, impair our judgment ("What am I doing here? Who is this guy?") and indeed decrease sexual response in 40 percent of those who use it. Chronic alcohol abuse is even worse, inhibiting desire and sexual functioning in anywhere from 23 to 100 percent of users. And when alcoholism causes liver damage, there can be subsequent hormonal and nerve changes that lead to arousal disorders. Alcohol affects sex and sex in turn affects alcoholism. The best predictor of whether an alcoholic woman will be able to stop drinking is her level of sexual dysfunction. In other words, some women who aren't getting pleasure from sex may be looking for satisfaction at the bottom of a bottle.

Finally, a word about caffeine: One of medical research's more fascinating findings is that people who drink more coffee (especially while listening to jazz) have more sex. But when caffeine intake and hormone levels were measured, it was found that high doses of caffeine (equivalent to more than two cups of coffee or four cans of caffeinated soda daily) raised levels of SHBG and, perhaps as a result, lowered levels of free testosterone. At least from a hormonal point of view, coffee may keep us up, but it won't help us get it up.

Approach to therapy: Don't inhale. But seriously, don't abuse drugs, alcohol—or even caffeine.

CHAPTER EIGHT

DISEASES

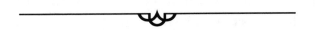

LONG-STANDING HEALTH PROBLEMS can make sex uncomfortable or difficult, alter our body's functions, cause depression and may distort our body image. The most common chronic conditions affecting sexual function are the following:

DIABETES

Despite the fact that 6 percent of women develop diabetes during their lifetime, the sexual problems of diabetic women were not even considered until 1970 (male impotence caused by diabetes had received major interest years before). The unfortunate fact is that up to one-third of women who become diabetic develop vaginal dryness and irritation and decreased genital sensitivity and may have diminished libido within four to six years after diagnosis.

Approach to therapy: Tight control of blood sugar will decrease the chance of nerve damage as well as the more immediate vaginal irritation caused by yeast infections. Intercourse may cause blood sugar levels to fall, which can be scary. Consider consuming a glass of orange juice or another sugar source before sex.

HEART AND LUNG DISEASES

These medical problems can make us so physically unfit that we're unable to muster our diminished reserves for intercourse; we are also afraid we'll exacerbate our condition (e.g., die of a heart attack) while having sex.

Approach to therapy: Many heart and lung medications may decrease desire independent of the disease, so work with your doctor to find substitutions that may have fewer sexual side effects. As for the fear of sex-induced heart attack: A study showed that only 0.9 percent of heart attacks occurred within two hours of sexual activity, and after some critical calculations it was decided that sex with your usual partner was extremely unlikely to land you in the cardiac ICU. The risk is even lower for those who exercise regularly. If you've had a heart attack, cardiac rehabilitation should help you perform all sorts of physical activities, including sex. The amount of exertion required for intercourse is roughly equivalent to climbing two flights of stairs, so if you can do the latter without chest pain you're probably physically fit enough to engage in the former, which is more fun.

CANCER

Despite the progress of science and medicine, the big C remains our greatest fear. And when a diagnosis confirms that fear, sex is probably the last thing we think about; we're too busy worrying about survival. But as we make decisions about surgery and chemotherapy, we need to weigh their potential effects on our sexuality.

Approach to therapy: For information on how cancer treatments can affect sexuality, see Chapter 9.

AUTOIMMUNE DISEASES

These sexist diseases—75 to 90 percent of cases occur in women—are caused by the body turning on itself and attacking its own tissues. One in 10 of us will develop an autoimmune disease during her lifetime. All these diseases can affect our sexuality.

SYSTEMIC LUPUS ERYTHEMATOSIS

Even women who are moderately ill with lupus are 26 percent less sexually active than average. They may have diminished vaginal lubrication, pain during intercourse, lower frequency of masturbation and greater depression. Corticosteroid drugs, one of the mainstays in the therapy for this disease, can cause weight gain which may contribute to poor body image.

RHEUMATOID ARTHRITIS

This disease causes joint deformity and pain, so finding a comfortable position to make love is a challenge.

SCLERODERMA

Overproduction of collagen causes scarring in our skin, internal organs and even the vulva and vagina. The latter can make sex uncomfortable.

SJOGRENS SYNDROME

Severe vaginal dryness and pain during intercourse are common complaints for women with this disease which dries tissues throughout the body. (One of my patients said that her vagina "felt like a prune" years before SS was finally diagnosed.)

THYROID DISEASE

Because this is usually an autoimmune disease, I've included it here. The thyroid is the mistress of our endocrine system and when it is not functioning properly, the effects are pan-glandular. Low thyroid hormone production (hypothyroidism) depresses our androgen levels and may be the unrecognized culprit behind male hormone inadequacy. Overproduction of thyroid hormone (hyperthyroidism, or Graves' disease) may also affect ovulation and ovarian hormones. This is why the thyroid should be tested whenever we suspect androgen deficiency. Measuring levels of thyroid-stimulating hormone (TSH) is the best way to determine if this "mama gland" is working properly.

MULTIPLE SCLEROSIS

This illness, which scars areas of the brain and spinal cord, can block genital enervation and diminish arousal and orgasm.

Approach to therapy: Try a vaginal moisturizer and use lubricants during intercourse if dryness is a problem. If you are menopausal, estrogen therapy may help. If you have joint pain, take an anti-inflammatory medication and a hot bath just before sex, and vary your sexual positions so you are more comfortable. Consider testosterone supplementation if a blood test shows levels are very low.

EPILEPSY

Women with epilepsy do not seem to have diminished sexual desire, but studies have found that more than one-third experience difficulty with arousal, pain during intercourse or vaginismus.

Approach to therapy: The problem is that the antilepileptic therapy, not the disease, may lower libido. You might ask your physician if you can switch from Tegretol to Depakote without sacrificing seizure control.

SPINAL CORD INJURIES

Because the nerves that control genital sexual response and sensation are often severed or damaged in spinal cord injuries, we would expect severe consequences for sexuality. The common misconception is that a woman who is paralyzed below the waist can't or won't want to have sex. But research shows that desire remains intact and these women can experience orgasm through fantasy and sexual contact. Sixty-nine percent of disabled women report that they are satisfied with their post-injury sexual experiences but not with the counseling about sex that they received after their injury.

Approach to therapy: Don't let anyone tell you that you can't continue to be sexual after a spinal cord injury. Viagra has helped men who have erection dysfunction after nerve injury. It's probable that it will also help women with similar arousal difficulties (see Chapter 11).

INCONTINENCE

If you leak urine when you cough or sneeze (stress incontinence), you are also more likely to leak during intercourse. This is probably because the opening of the bladder moves down and out in response to abdominal pressure during penetration. Even women who don't have stress incontinence may have the embarrassing problem of losing urine during orgasm. Nerves that trigger involuntary contractions of the bladder run through the same pathway as those that mediate sexual response, and their stimulation can lead to both orgasm and loss of urine.

Relaxation of our pelvic muscles is a price we often pay for vaginal deliveries. When the bladder is bulging from the vagina (cystocele) or the rectum is bulging (rectocele), or when everything comes down so that the cervix and part of the uterus are in the lower third of the vagina (pelvic prolapse), we can experience discomfort and pressure during intercourse. Between 34 and 45 percent of women with any form of pelvic prolapse are incontinent during sex.

Approach to therapy: Emptying the bladder just prior to intercourse should help prevent incontinence. Antispasmodic drugs such as Ditropan or Urispas, which stop bladder contractions, can be taken two hours before sex to control involuntary loss of urine. For prolapse, consider using vaginal support devices, or pessaries, during the day to keep the organs in place and removing them just prior to intercourse; also use vaginal estrogen to keep the tissue healthy and lubricated. If these methods aren't enough, surgery to put the protruding organs back in their proper place, or even vaginal hysterectomy, may be the only solution.

STDS

Sexually transmitted diseases range from those that barely cause symptoms to ones that are devastating and can end our lives. Their effect on our sexuality is practically always negative, either because we are afraid of getting or giving an STD during intercourse or because its presence causes irritation, discharge and/or painful lesions.

STDs may turn out to be our ultimate modern libido killer. In the last decade, I have found that many more of my patients are abstaining from sexual activity because of distrust and fear of contracting an STD. They have gotten so accustomed to their celibate condition that they've actually forgotten how great sex can be. They have lost touch with their fantasies, their need for intimacy and themselves (literally).

Approach to therapy: Masturbation is safe sex and will help us maintain our awareness of the pleasure that our body can give. Although condoms are not foolproof or germ-proof, they will certainly limit our chances of becoming infected, as will choosing a partner who is low-risk and who has tested negative for HIV.

CHAPTER NINE

SURGERY, CHEMOTHERAPY AND RADIATION

M ANY OF THE MEDICAL PROCEDURES associated with the treatment of pelvic disease and cancer can trigger sudden menopause with disastrous libido results. When our ovaries are surgically removed or destroyed by radiation or chemotherapy, the resultant hormonal shock to our body is enormous. If we are not already menopausal, we suddenly lose our major source of estrogen, progesterone and at least half of our testosterone. So in addition to dealing with the subsequent and usually severe hot flashes, sleep disturbances, depression, vaginal dryness, weight changes, memory loss and lack of periods, we're losing the sense of desire for and enjoyment of the sexual intimacy that could help us cope with all of the above. Our loss of reproductive capability (especially at an early age) can mean that lovemaking evokes a sense of grief instead of one of joy. Although chemotherapy, radiation and surgery cause the same hormonal results, each has its own side effects, so let's look at them separately.

CHEMOTHERAPY

Fatigue, lethargy, depression, nausea, vomiting, hair loss and weight gain are common side effects of chemotherapy. Fortunately, they are all temporary. But while they are happening, sex gets put on the back burner. The real damage to our libido comes from chemotherapy's chemical shutdown of our ovaries, which, if a woman is over age 35, may turn out to be permanent. (Younger women may get a return of ovarian functions but later are at risk for early menopause.) The immediate effects of chemotherapy on sexual response will be due to sudden loss of estrogen and testosterone. Estrogen deprivation will prevent pelvic and vaginal congestion and lubrication, so arousal becomes difficult if not impossible. But the real libido saboteur is loss of testosterone, which robs us of clitoral sensation and depresses desire, fantasy, orgasm and pleasure. We feel "chem-oed" from the waist down.

RADIATION THERAPY

When radiation to the abdomen or pelvis causes loss of ovarian function, it will ultimately have the same effect as chemotherapy. It can also cause scarring and shortening of the vagina.

REMOVAL OF BOTH OVARIES

This procedure, called bilateral oophorectomy, may be performed alone to treat benign disease or early ovarian malignancies or to prevent ovarian cancer. It can also be combined with hysterectomy (removal of the uterus) for the treatment of pelvic cancers or benign diseases such as endometriosis, pelvic adhesions (scar tissue), cysts or fibroids. There has been a decidedly cavalier "we're there anyway, let's take them out—you never know what might happen in the fu-

SEX AFTER CHEMOTHERAPY

Sally is a physician who first consulted me at the age of 41 because she was having irregular cycles. She hadn't had a mammogram for two years. Her hormone levels were fine, but I felt a nodule in her right breast. Tests showed that the lump was cancerous, and because of its size she opted for a mastectomy. Six of her lymph nodes contained malignant cells, and Sally then had extensive chemotherapy and a bone marrow transplant. She pulled through, but was left completely menopausal with severe hot flashes, vaginal dryness, insomnia and no libido. Sex was very painful. When she attempted to use Tamoxifen (an anti-estrogen that can decrease breast cancer recurrence), her symptoms got worse and she stopped after six months. For the next five years, she coped, trying vaginal lubricants, herbs and exercise. She eventually stopped having sex.

On her five-year cancer-free anniversary, Sally decided that after making it this far without a recurrence she wanted the quality of her life restored. We had a long talk and she opted to start with a very low-dose estrogen patch (Fem-Patch), a vaginal estrogen ring (Estring) and methyltestosterone lozenges, or troches, (0.5 milligrams daily under her tongue). To protect her uterus, she also started taking natural progesterone: 100 milligrams nightly.

Sally is ecstatic about the results and, yes, her libido has returned. She has been my most informed consumer, reading all of the medical literature on the pros and cons of estrogen therapy after breast cancer. Currently it seems that there is no documented increase in recurrence rates, metastases or mortality in women who take estrogen after breast cancer as compared to similar women who don't. Sally also learned about testosterone metabolism. Knowing all this, she decided to take advantage of what hormones have to offer. She is very realistic about her future risks, but right now, she feels she has got it up—her life, her health and her sexuality.

ture" attitude toward our ovaries. As a result, 68 percent of women over the age of 45 are having their ovaries removed at the time of hysterectomy. Most of our post-hysterectomy complaints and our dissatisfaction with its effect on our libido should really be directed at the ovarian portion of the surgery!

The same acute hormonal deficiency seen with chemotherapy will obviously be present with surgery, but if anything, will occur more quickly (within 24 to 48 hours) and be more intense. A study of women who underwent oopherectomy without estrogen replacement therapy showed that they had significantly more body image problems than did women who had the same surgery and were given estrogen or who "just" had a hysterectomy. Loss of our ovaries and hormones can be a truly defeminizing event—perhaps even greater than the loss of our womb.

Approach to therapy: Our ovaries can continue to produce male hormone years after menopause, and the offhand recommendation that we have healthy ovaries removed just because we're near "that age" needs to be revisited. Informed consent is incomplete if the impact of our surgical choices on our libido has not been addressed.

Estrogen replacement after ovarian removal or destruction depends on the nature of the underlying disease. In the absence of cancer, estrogen should be started right away, before the symptoms of hormone withdrawal become severe. (When I perform a bilateral oopherectomy, I immediately apply an estrogen patch in the O.R.) The concept of testosterone replacement is new, although the symptoms of testosterone withdrawal have always been there. But the same principles should apply and immediate testosterone therapy should be considered.

If the surgery was done for cancer and either you or your physician are hesitant about starting hormone replacement therapy, local estrogen creams or a vaginal estrogen ring (Estring) will certainly help alleviate vaginal dryness and painful intercourse. (Please note: There is still a very small absorption of estrogen into the bloodstream.) Local testosterone ointment or cream may also help and methyltestosterone troches (lozenges placed under the tongue), which undergo less conversion to estrogen than "pure" testosterone, have become an additional option (see Chapter 12). In the future we may also prescribe medications such as Viagra (see Chapter 11).

HYSTERECTOMY

The problem: A near-religious belief in the potency of the uterus has been with us since the days (and nights) of Cleopatra. Even in modern times there are believers and heretics. One-third of women will have a hysterectomy by age 60, so it's important that we consider the reasons for the devoted opinions of each group. How important is the uterus to our psychological and sexual well-being? If we are to believe the believers (chiefly European physicians), the cervix and uterus play a critical role in the quality of orgasm. Pressure on the cervix as well as contractions of the uterus may be part of women's sexual response. (The anatomists proclaim the importance of the nerve fibers around the cervix and have even given these fibers a great name: the plexus of Frankenhauser.) The pro-cervical faction also points out that removal of the cervix can shorten the vagina, making intercourse uncomfortable. This camp states that there is in addition a higher rate of subsequent prolapse of the top of the vagina when the cervix is removed. They theorize that psychologically, loss of these organs diminishes sexual pleasure and may lead women to mourn the loss of their reproductive soul.

The heretics (mostly Americans) discount the sexual input of the cervix and note that when it is removed, the future risk of cervical cancer is eliminated. They also point out that a hysterectomy is done for reasons such as pelvic pain and heavy bleeding, and that relieving these problems will, if anything, improve depression and sexual response. They proclaim that women who have hysterectomies start out with more psychological problems and so if there are problems after, the surgery can't be blamed.

So much for religion. What do the studies show? Canadian research done on three groups of women having hysterectomy, tubal ligation or removal of their gallbladder showed no significant differences between the groups when it came to postsurgery depression or anxiety. Three other studies looked at sexual response after total hysterectomy (removal of the uterus and cervix but not the ovaries), and found that two-thirds of the women had the same or an improved response after surgery and that one-third felt worse. (Perhaps this third was comprised of women for whom cervical and uterine stimulation played an important part in orgasm.)

Everyone agrees that if sex was good before hysterectomy, it is less likely to diminish afterward. It may even improve if the surgery puts an end to pelvic pain and heavy bleeding.

Approach to therapy: Once more, your informed consent has to deal with the sexual implications of surgery. There does appear to be a group of women who are conscious of the orgasmic contribution of their cervix and uterus, and your personal assessment of what gives you pleasure should help guide your decision. The mode of surgery may also make a difference. Vaginal hysterectomy (done without an abdominal incision) cannot be performed without removal of the cervix. This surgery has a shorter, less painful recovery period than an abdominal approach, and from personal experience I know that many of my patients would trade their cervix for an easy, speedy recovery.

BREAST SURGERY

Breast cancer is potentially devastating to a woman's self-image and sexual function. Up to 30 percent of women who have had it report a decrease in their frequency of intercourse or ability to orgasm; however, it appears that the greatest damage to their sexual pleasure comes from the chemotherapy that is so frequently part of their treatment.

The surgical debate vis-à-vis libido is over whether conservative surgery (lumpectomy) will better conserve our sexual response than mastectomy, and whether mastectomy should be followed by breast reconstruction. Women who undergo lumpectomies or who have their breast(s) reconstructed after mastectomy rate their body image more highly and are more comfortable with nudity and breast caressing than women who have had mastectomies without reconstruction. In addition, those who have both their breast and nipple reconstructed are happier with erotic sensation than those who have only breast mounds. Choice is important, and women who have been allowed to decide between lumpectomy and mastectomy have been found to be less depressed one year after surgery than women who were told what they had to do (or woke up with it done).

Breast surgery may have more severe emotional consequences for younger women. Those who have no current partner face the fear of telling a new lover that they have had cancer and then exposing the evidence. They must also deal with the fact that chemotherapy may preclude future childbearing. Even among women over age 40, those who are in their forties and early fifties rate mastectomy as more negative to their sexual relationship than older women. Despite all this, we have remarkable recuperative powers. Research shows that no matter what a woman's age, ultimately the health of her relationship, her psyche and her sex life does not differ significantly whether she has a mastectomy or lumpectomy.

Approach to therapy: For most of us, our future survival is far more important than the survival of our breast, and the surgery that will give us the best chance of beating this disease is the one we want. Seventy percent of all breast cancers can be as successfully treated with lumpectomy and radiation as with mastectomy. If you fall into that 70 percent, know that you have a choice and that you should be the one to make it. The more comfortable you are with your decision, the more comfortable you will be with your body and your sexuality.

CHAPTER TEN

PAIN

Nothing diminishes our desire to have sex like pain. The pain can be anywhere in our body, and pain from the neck up has evolved into the motto of diminished libido, "Not tonight, honey, I have a headache." But it is just as valid to substitute joint pain, back pain, abdominal pain and chest pain (for the last we should be going to the emergency room, not to bed). In any case, the approach to therapy is to discover the cause and treat the discomfort.

Another more local pain that can have major consequences on our sexual functioning and libido is that which occurs during intercourse. The medical profession must have recognized the importance of this pain, because they gave it its own name: dyspareunia. This is the most common sexual complaint reported to gynecologists, and surveys have shown that it occurs in 10 to 15 percent of women. Dyspareunia is often caused by physical problems, but many doctors dismiss it as an "all in your head" condition because they can't see that anything is wrong. However, there is something physically wrong in 76 percent of women who are suffering from this condition. It might be vaginal infection, estrogen deprivation, muscle spasm (vaginismus) or chronic inflammation of glands surrounding the lower part of the opening of the vagina (vestibulitis). Or it could be a bladder or urethral infection, pelvic inflammatory disease (PID), endometriosis or other pelvic pathology. Relationship conflict or past sexual abuse may also be a contributing factor. Let's consider some of these physical causes in more detail.

VULVODYNIA

This is defined as an extraordinary sensitivity anywhere in the vulva but most often in the lower part of the vagina near the entrance (the vestibulum). Touch or pressure in this area, during either penetration or an exam, elicits a burning, stinging pain or sense of rawness. The area can appear redder than the rest of the vagina and touching it, even with a Q-tip, often elicits an extreme reaction. Although we don't know what causes vulvodynia, it has been linked with multiple irritating factors such as yeast infection, use of antibiotics and antibiotic creams, cryosurgery or laser surgery. Vulvodynia seems to occur more frequently in women who have irritable bowel syndrome or interstitial cystitis (a chronic inflammation of the bladder). In the past doctors thought the human papillomavirus (HPV) and microscopic genital warts might be responsible, but this link has never been proven and HPV therapy won't ease the pain.

Approach to therapy: We start from the benign and proceed to the extreme. Vitamin A and D ointment, 1 percent hydrocortisone ointment (not cream—it contains alcohol and will burn like crazy!), 2 percent lidocaine gel and 1,000 to 2,000 milligrams of calcium twice a day have all been reported to work. If none of these help, tricyclic antidepressants and lithium can be tried. And if these fail, surgery to remove the sensitive tissue of the vestibulum works 80 percent of the time.

Once we stop having sex because it hurts, we remember the hurt and avoid reliving it, sometimes even after the source of the pain is gone. In deference to this, it may be necessary to combine psychotherapy or sex therapy with treatments for longstanding physical complaints.

LOCALIZED PAIN

Jenny is a 23-year-old single woman who works as an administrative assistant. She became sexually active three years ago, but every time she had intercourse, she experienced pain in one defined and unchanging spot at the entrance of her vagina. This became so severe that she started to dread sex or even touching in her genital area. The result was inevitable—her boyfriend "uncommitted" to the relationship, and she was afraid to start a new one. Jenny went from doctor to doctor in search of a cure. She was treated for possible yeast infections, bacterial infections, herpes and dermatitis; nothing worked.

When I examined her, I saw nothing. But when I touched the sensitive area with a Q-tip, I elicited a big "Ouch!" After much discussion, we decided to take a fairly radical approach (after all, she had tried everything else): I would surgically remove the affected region of the inner labia and vestibulum. This can help relieve localized pain if the nerve endings are overly sensitized or have formed an abnormal growth called a neuroma. Jenny decided that she would need a general anesthetic to go through with it, so I performed this surgery in our outpatient department at the hospital. Once she was under anesthesia, I outlined the area with a pen and as I did so, I heard the anesthesiologist exclaim, "Wow, that must really hurt." Her heartbeat had quickened only when I touched the sensitive region. The surgery went well and, remarkably, Jenny had very little pain as she healed. Six weeks later, I could apply Q-tips, direct pressure, and pull on the area with a speculum, without causing discomfort.

I got a call from Jenny six months later. She met this great guy, and they had sex. It didn't hurt!

VAGINISMUS

This involuntary spasm of the outer musculature of the vagina has been found to occur in 12 to 17 percent of women requesting treatment at sex therapy clinics. It can be primary (there from the start) or secondary (occuring later in life). It is universal when an attempt to insert anything—a finger, a tampon, a speculum or a penis—into the vagina elicits spasm. Or it can be situational, occurring solely during attempts at sexual penetration. Psychological issues such as a strict antisexual upbringing, sex fears and phobias and a history of abuse or trauma probably have a greater role in this diagnosis than in any other cause of dyspareunia.

Approach to therapy: Desensitization of the area. Either the patient or, if she is willing, her partner can begin this gradual process by inserting fingers followed by tampons and special dilators into the vagina, and finally attempting intercourse. There is an 80 percent success rate in couples where the partner is involved.

OTHER FORMS AND CAUSES OF DYSPAREUNIA

For diagnosis and treatment of the problem, you have to be very graphic in describing your symptoms while your doctor uses her or his acumen to assess the physical signs.

- *If the pain is accompanied by itching, burning or stinging* and is made worse by the initiation of penetration, it may be due to a yeast infection or inflammation of the vulva, in which case local medication will take care of the problem. In the absence of infection, your doctor might want to do a biopsy to detect abnormal changes in the cells of the vulva, some of which could be precancerous. Biopsy often reveals a condition called Lichen Sclerosis et Atrophicus, which has traditionally been treated with testosterone ointment. This disorder has historic significance because women who were treated with testosterone ointment remarked that it increased their clitoral sensitivity, arousal and libido. This therapy was ultimately not as successful a treatment as the potent steroid cream clobetasol, but we may have this condition and those women to thank for discovery of the sexual benefits of local testosterone therapy.

- *If the pain occurs only during deep thrusting* and you have the sensation that your partner is "bumping into" something, it may be caused by endometriosis, pelvic adhesions, uterine fibroids or ovarian cysts. Your doctor should check for these and treat you accordingly. One-third of us have a uterus that is tilted down toward the base of our spine (retroverted), and when the penis pushes the uterus back into the pelvis where there is little room we may get cramps or pain. The solution is simple: Change the direction of thrust by being on top or lying on your stomach.

- *Feelings of tightness* (he doesn't "fit") may be due to spasm or postoperative narrowing, but in some cases, with very tall or well-endowed partners, there truly is a size problem.

- *Tenderness of the bladder*, which may cause you to feel like you need to void, can be due to bladder or urethral infections or, on occasion, a cyst or pocket (called a diverticulum) in the urethra. Many women find that sex causes recurrent bladder infections and benefit from better "bladder hygiene," which includes drinking plenty of water, taking cranberry tablets (found in health food stores), urinating before and after intercourse and sometimes taking an antibiotic right after sexual activity.

- *That "sandpaper" feeling,* when friction during intercourse makes you feel as though the vaginal walls are tearing, is due to inadequate lubrication during arousal. The most common cause is estrogen deficiency, which obviously makes estrogen the solution (for details on your treatment options, see chapters 12 and 13). Some women notice an increase in dryness after they begin taking oral contraceptives; this may improve if they switch to a birth control pill that has more estrogen. Masturbation and frequent intercourse is one more therapy of choice for vaginal dryness and atrophy!

CHAPTER ELEVEN

THE SEVENTH SABOTEUR: MEN

I F WE DON'T HAVE A PARTNER, or if the partner we have can't or won't participate in a satisfactory sexual union, we lose an important opportunity to be "in the mood." The 20 million American men who suffer from impotence may constitute our greatest sexual problem. Even the National Institutes of Health has attacked the issue in a consensus conference on men (there seemed to be a consensus that female sexual dysfunction didn't rate a conference). They informed us that the word "impotence" was pejorative and should no longer be used to define a man's lack of ability to have or maintain a firm erection. Instead, we should use the more precise term, "erectile dysfunction," to signify "an inability of the male to achieve an erect penis as part of the overall multifaceted process of male sexual function." The sad news about this politically correct term is that it is broader (no pun intended) and encompasses partial erectile dysfunction as well as total failure. This means the number of our erectilly challenged partners rises to 30 million!

The older your partner, the more likely he will have erectile dysfunction. Between the ages of 20 and 30, it occurs in 5 to 7 percent of the male population, but it affects more than 25 percent of men over age 65. At the age of 70, the number goes up to 50 percent. No matter when it occurs, even if the failure is partial (meaning it doesn't happen all the time or result in complete loss of rigidity), erectile dysfunction often causes men to fear future failure and become unwilling to initiate intercourse. The underlying reasons (as with our female erectile dysfunction) are classified as psychological or medical.

PSYCHOLOGICAL FACTORS

Psychological troubles that lead to male erectile dysfunction are similar to those that diminish our arousal response and include depression, anxiety, stress and relationship problems. All of these reduce a man's ability to focus on erotic sensations and hamper his awareness of sex as a sensory experience. Men, unlike women, are going to manifest their reduced erotic focus in a very obvious way. They can't fake an erection. Since seeing is believing, the psychiatric world has a final result on which to focus its attention.

MEDICAL FACTORS

Medical problems that cause erectile difficulties include any diseases or medications that impair blood flow to the penis or damage the pathways of nerves to or from this organ. The diseases are multiple and common: diabetes, hypertension, coronary vascular disease, peripheral vascular disorders such as arteriosclerosis, and neurological conditions. Fifty percent of diabetic men will experience some erectile dysfunction within five years of their diagnosis, probably because the disease affects both the blood vessels and nerves. Men who have arteriosclerosis that involves their coronary vessels generally have the same problem in their penile arteries. It is interesting to note that one study, which compared two groups of men with heart disease, showed that if they couldn't have an erection, they were more likely to have a heart attack in the future. The functioning of their penile vessels predicted or even mirrored the functioning of their coronary vessels (my first scientific documentation that the hearts of men are ruled by their . . .).

SURGICAL FACTORS

The commonly performed surgery used to treat an enlarged prostate gland, transurethral resection of the prostate (TURP), may result in a 4 to 20 percent rate of erectile dysfunction. More radical abdominal surgery done for prostate cancer has an extremely high rate of trauma to the nerves and blood supply, with the subsequent loss of ability to have an erection.

HORMONAL FACTORS

Just like women, men can have a deficiency of testosterone (I've been waiting throughout this entire book to give you my reverse take on a traditionally male-oriented statement), so the work-up of male sexual dysfunction should include a testosterone blood test. If the level is low, replacement should be prescribed. This is certainly not a problem, because most testosterone pills, shots and patches have been tailored for male hormonal needs.

PHARMACEUTICAL FACTORS

The medications that lower our female sexual arousal and drive can do the same to men. Chief among them (because so many men end up taking them) are medications that treat high blood pressure or heart disease. Then, of course, there are the antidepressants, antipsychotics and anti-anxiety medications. Steroid abuse by body builders, illicit drug abuse, alcohol and smoking, which constrict vessels that supply the penis, can all cause erectile problems.

AGING

Basic physiological and sexual function changes over the years may be inevitable, and these include:

- Reduced free testosterone levels (not quite the equivalent of our menopause, but still a relative "testosterone pause")
- Reduced size and volume of the testes
- Increased size and volume of the prostate gland
- Decrease in the number and frequency of morning erections
- Slower response to visual and nongenital stimulation
- More dependence on manual stimulation to attain erection
- Poorly defined sense of impending orgasm
- Decreased strength of genital muscle spasm with orgasm
- Decreased ejaculatory force
- Reduced viscosity and volume of semen
- Rapid return to a non-erectile state (detumescence)
- Longer delay until they can do it again (refractory period)

Since erectile dysfunction increases so substantially with age, should we expect the older men in our lives to be able to continue their role and partnership in our sexual activity? Yes, but they may have to work at it. They have to maintain their physical well-being. The better their cardiovascular condition, the lower their cholesterol and the better their lung capacity, the less likely they will become erectilly challenged. So when it comes to sexual maintenance, the old rules apply: Exercise, eat right, don't get fat and don't smoke. If our partners do begin to have problems, it behooves us to be understanding and patient, and to participate in their attempts to get help. If they sense that we're angry or disgusted or feel they are inadequate, it will only fuel their performance fear and become a psychological factor. A man's libido is a fragile thing.

Approach to therapy: Treatment obviously has to include a medical work-up to look for chronic illness and a thorough search for possible causes of erectile dysfunction such as medication, alcohol or drug abuse and hormonal deficiency, as well as psychological issues. Once diagnosed, the disease should be treated, the erectile and libido-affecting medications changed and/or the psychological problems addressed by a trained professional (see Chapter 14). If testosterone deficiency is found, a testosterone patch can be worn on the testes to give a sort of "express delivery" to the end organ, or it can be applied to skin elsewhere on the body. These won't work in men with normal testosterone levels.

Then there are the therapies that are specifically designed to cause erection—shots, pills and implants. Here is a brief discussion of each.

INJECTION THERAPY

The biochemistry of erection has attracted considerable research and produced subsequent results. In 1995, scientists developed alprostadil, a natural substance (prostaglandin E-1) normally present in penile arteries. When released, it relaxes smooth muscle cells, allowing the arteries to fill with blood. The initial product was called Caverjet and was injected into the side of the penis near the base, about 20 minutes before sex. It created an erection that lasted an hour or more. Another formulation called Edex came out in 1997 and was delivered with a smaller needle. Alprostadil was also supplied as a suppository that could be inserted into the tip of the penis; it was called the

Muse Pellet (I'm only reporting this and make no comment on how pharmaceutical companies come up with product names). It could be used twice a day and worked 10 minutes after application. You may notice that I've used the past tense for all of these products; you will understand why when you get to the section on pills below.

VACUUM CONSTRICTIVE DEVICES

These push blood into the penis, but certainly limit spontaneity (which probably has been lost with all of these therapies) and may cause "some discomfort" (I'm cringing at the description).

PENILE IMPLANTS

These are surgically implanted and can be inflated or are manually (or womanully) operated.

PILLS

Viagra (sildenafil), the new oral preparation for erectile dysfunction, is making Pfizer's stockholders' dreams come true. It should also make implementation of the sexual dreams of tens of millions of men and their partners come true. Viagra works by blocking an enzyme that breaks down cyclic guanosine monophosphate (GMP). This substance is normally released during sexual stimulation and causes smooth muscle cells surrounding the erectile arteries in the penis to relax so that the arteries become engorged. If the breakdown enzyme is blocked, the levels of cyclic GMP rise and stay up (quantitatively and physiologically). Viagra has no effect in the absence of sexual stimulation, so it doesn't cause an unheeded erection. If taken 30 to 120 minutes before stimulation, the right dose facilitates the response of the vessels so that they fill up in 80 to 88 percent of men with erectile dysfunction. This response is strong enough to allow 69 percent to have successful intercourse. Improvement was noted, albeit at lower rates, even after nerve damage from spinal injury or radical prostate surgery, as well as in men with medical problems such as diabetes and cardiac and vascular disease. In tests, Viagra also helped patients taking antidepressants, antipsychotics or antihypertensive medication. Most side effects were considered to be minor, or at least worth it. They included headache, flushing, runny nose, stomach upset and blue vision in 6 to 30 percent of the men. The most prevalent problem was headache, which might result in the advice: Take an aspirin, a Viagra and go to bed . . . But, putting Viagra jokes aside, the much more adverse reactions of heart attack, stroke and death have now been reported as millions of men have used this drug. Since Viagra affects nitric oxide production (this is what stimulates GMP) and can lower blood pressure, it's dangerous to combine it with heart medications that contain nitrates such as nitroglycerine or blood pressure–lowering drugs. There are also concerns about reactions in men taking Glucatrol, a diabetes drug.

Despite these warnings, it appears that this is indeed a "V for victory" drug. Pfizer reported that Viagra improved "frequency, firmness, and maintenance of erection; frequency of orgasm; frequency and level of desire; frequency satisfaction; enjoyment of intercourse and overall relationship satisfaction" in men who had previous erectile dysfunction. Theoretically, Viagra should have no effect on desire, but I guess if the plumbing works, these men will want to use it. The drug is not supposed to cause "super"-erections, nor improve the performance of men whose erections are normal. If they produce enough cyclic GMP, they don't need more. But there are anecdotal reports that erections last longer and that refractory time is shortened or eliminated when Viagra is used.

So now that individuals possessing an XY chromosome have received help in pill form, what about us? Clearly, if our sexual saboteur is an erectilly dysfunctional male partner, we have just been given a major sexual boost. But Viagra and future generations of similar drugs should also be able to boost our own erections, triggering vaginal and clitoral response. Shouldn't we share? Testing is now being conducted to assess the response and appropriate doses in women. Until we have the results of this testing, we can enjoy sharing in our partners' ability to have intercourse. In the near future, we should be able to share their pills or have our very own.

PART THREE

THE
LIBIDINOUS
SOLUTIONS

CHAPTER TWELVE

TESTOSTERONE AND BEYOND:

Our Newest Hormone Replacement Options

Not only has the study of sexual dysfunction traditionally ignored women, but the study of male hormones and their effect on sexual dysfunction has continued this gender bias. A man who can't have an erection because of low testosterone levels is an endocrinologic catastrophe, whereas an androgen-deficient woman is much harder to recognize and falls into the category of "oh well, you don't need it anyway."

When traditional medicine deigned to look at androgens in women, it was only to examine and bemoan the unfortunate physical consequences of too much testosterone. So let's acknowledge tradition and begin this section with an overview of androgen excess.

Five to 10 percent of women have a condition called polycystic ovarian syndrome (PCO), in which the ovaries and/or adrenal glands produce too much male hormone. This hormonal disturbance usually begins at puberty and is accompanied by excess hair growth, irregular menstrual cycles and obesity. Those of us affected subsequently may be infertile and are at high risk for diabetes, hypertension and heart disease as well as uterine and breast cancer. This syndrome is too complex to describe in detail in this book (I'd have to write another one), but suffice it to say that the latest theories suggest that PCO is often linked to an inability of the body to let insulin do its job (a condition called insulin resistance). When the naysayers point to this syndrome and say, "Egad, look what male hormones can do," they are comparing apples (male-pattern weight distribution common in women with PCO) with pears (the typical female pattern). Very rarely, conditions of excess male hormone production can develop later in life from tumors of the ovaries or adrenal glands, or Cushing's syndrome.

The far more common scenario is that at some point in our lives, most of us will become testosterone deficient. Between our twenties and forties, our circulating testosterone declines by 50 percent. Then, with the onset of menopause, it drops an additional 30 to 50 percent (see Chapter 3). This can be accompanied by diminished sexual desire and arousability, inability to climax, loss of pubic hair, skin thinning and an overall diminished sense of well-being. For hundreds of years we have remained hapless victims of estrogen loss, and have finally spent the last few decades investigating whether it is worthwhile to replace estrogen after menopause. Hormone replacement therapy has been a godsend to many women (although God didn't send it, the pharmaceutical companies did). We are now at the threshold of a similar revolution when it comes to male hormones.

TESTOSTERONE THERAPY: THE GOOD NEWS

Most of what we know about the effects of testosterone supplementation comes from studies of women whose ovaries were surgically removed; the rest of our information comes from research done with naturally menopausal women. Since the majority of these women were divided into groups that were treated with estrogen alone, estrogen and testosterone or a placebo, it is difficult to make claims about the effects of treatment with testosterone alone. Once estrogen is factored out of the equation, however, testosterone appears to do the following:

Boost desire. At least 10 studies have specifically examined testosterone's effect on libido, and still others have noted a link. When the different stages of our sexual response were examined, the general consensus was that testosterone caused a decrease in sexual inhibition and an increase in motivation, arousal and fantasy (which together equal libido). Researchers also reported an increase in orgasmic intensity. The findings are not as clear when it comes to whether testosterone affects frequency of intercourse. Some say yes; others say it makes no difference. In any case, quality is probably more important than quantity.

Increase psychological well-being. Studies using a variety of different formulations of testosterone at varying dosages (some of them extremely high) have reported an overall improvement in practically every facet of our psyches, and frankly this sounds too good to be true. These include (smile when you read this) increased energy and less fatigue; a sense of being composed or elated; increased ability to concentrate; decreased depression, nervousness, irritability and insomnia; and, finally, an improved sense of well-being. One study even reported that women given male hormone improved their scores on math problem solving and spatial functioning. (The researchers went on to say that basic differences in testosterone levels may explain why males score better than we do on math tests.) In a few studies, there was one other finding that most of us won't consider a huge advantage: increased appetite.

Strengthen our bones. Our bones have both estrogen and androgen receptors. The increase in androgen during puberty is felt to be partly responsible for our growth spurt. Bone is constantly being broken down and rebuilt throughout our lives. Androgens help the building part of this process and consequently might protect against osteoporosis. All the studies examining bone density involved estrogen, which we know prevents osteoporosis, so adding testosterone was not earth- (or bone-) shattering. But some investigators found that the increase in spinal bone density was twice as high in women who took both estrogen and testosterone as in women who took estrogen alone.

Ease rheumatoid arthritis. Androgens may be natural immune suppressors. Women, who have one-tenth the amount of testosterone that men have, are three times as likely to develop rheumatoid arthritis (RA). I doubt this is a simple coincidence. It has been shown that women who develop RA have lower testosterone levels than those who do not, and one study found that when women with the disease were given testosterone for one year, 21 percent showed improvement in their painful symptoms, versus only 4 percent of women given a placebo.

Improve menopausal symptoms. Although estrogen does a fabulous job diminishing hot flashes, night sweats, insomnia, vaginal dryness and other menopausal symptoms, sometimes it just isn't enough. Adding testosterone improves on these results for women who don't respond adequately to estrogen alone. It may also offset one of estrogen's annoying and scary side effects: breast tenderness.

DOES TESTOSTERONE HAVE
A DARK SIDE?

COSMETIC CONCERNS

The trepidation for many women (and yes, their doctors) is that taking testosterone will turn them into hairy, pimply, aggressive monsters with an enlarged clitoris and a deep voice. Not a pretty image, but not an accurate one either. Unlike pharmacological doses (which can result in blood levels that are many times greater than what we produce in our reproductive years), physiological doses (those meant to mimic the body's natural production of male hormone) won't do this. In a study in which acne and excess hair growth (hirsutism) on the face, abdomen, breasts and back were noted, the women were given 10 times the amount of testosterone their bodies would naturally make. The same goes for enlargement of the clitoris (clitoromegaly). And the fact that this clitoromegaly did not go away when the women stopped taking the hormone has been used ad nauseum to scare us out of taking testosterone altogether.

This is not to say that testosterone in lower doses can't cause some degree of acne, facial hair growth or male pattern balding. Studies that looked at these possible problems were carried out on women who took a pill that combined estrogen and synthetic testosterone (Estratest). Two strengths were used, and side effects appear to be hairier and scarier in those who took the larger dose. In one two-year study of the higher-dose pill, there was a 36 percent increase in hirsutism and acne, although the researchers assured us that it wasn't severe. (Most of us are plucking hairs as we get older without testosterone supplementation.) A study of the lower-dose pill was conducted on only 26 women, and among the 13 who took it for six months, there were five reports of acne and two reports of facial hair.

However, one woman in the estrogen-only group also complained of facial hair. The dreaded, permanent clitoromegaly was not seen in women who took the higher-dose pill in another two-year study.

CHOLESTEROL AND CARDIOVASCULAR CONSIDERATIONS

Cardiovascular disease is the leading cause of death for American women. We are valiantly struggling to overcome this and certainly don't want to make matters worse (although smoking, obesity and lack of exercise, which are endemic to our society, have certainly eroded our efforts). Most heart attacks are due to atherosclerosis, in which cholesterol plaques block our vessels. This process is linked to increased levels of cholesterol, especially "bad" or "sticky" low density lipoprotein (LDL) cholesterol. Both total cholesterol and LDL levels, as well as levels of another nasty blood fat, triglycerides, rise rapidly after menopause, one of the reasons that heart disease in women increases tenfold after this transition. But not all cholesterol is bad. High density lipoprotein (HDL) cholesterol prevents fat globules from being deposited on the walls of our vessels and even helps scrape some globules off—a combined Teflon and Drano effect.

So much for lipid chemistry. Studies overwhelmingly show that taking estrogen after menopause reduces our risk of heart disease. One of the ways it does this is by lowering total cholesterol; moreover, it improves the ratio of HDL to LDL, raising HDL levels and lowering LDL. Please note that LDL has now been subdivided, and the very low density lipoprotein component, or VLDL, is the worst instigator of plaque formation. This too is lowered by estrogen. But these lipid effects account for only 25 percent of estrogen's heart-healthy effort on our behalf. The other 75 percent has to do with estrogen's direct impact on our blood vessels and heart, where it relaxes arteries, increases blood flow to the heart, improves heart muscle contraction, lowers blood pressure and makes platelets less sticky so clots don't form.

The question is, does adding male hormone to our estrogen replacement diminish our cardiac protection? The answer, as usual, is murky. It appears from most studies that the addition of testosterone decreases total cholesterol (so far, so good), while decreasing the good HDL (bad), decreasing LDL and VLDL (good) and finally decreasing triglycerides (also good). So how does this add up? It depends on whether the final analysis is being made in Europe or the United States. Americans are great cholesterol believers and feel that estrogen protection of our hearts comes from the changes made in cholesterol. The Europeans are more likely to blame triglycerides for heart attacks in women and heartily believe that anything that will lower triglycerides is good for our coronary arteries.

We may lose a little HDL, but we gain a little in the triglyceride arena (and triglycerides increasingly are being seen as a key factor in heart attacks in women). Moreover, even though HDL is lowered, for most women it remains in the normal range, especially when low doses of testosterone are used. But all these lipid changes are just the results of blood tests, and how they translate into our real world of heart disease and heart attacks is not yet known.

So our lipids are left with a few pluses and a few minuses when we add testosterone to estrogen. What about the other 75 percent of estrogen's cardioprotective effects? Our only studies here were conducted on monkeys, and testosterone did not block estrogen's benefits to their blood vessels or heart. So can we extrapolate that what's good for a monkey heart is good for our hearts? I don't have the heart to make that decision. The long-term effects of testosterone on our cardiac status is still unknown. Each of us will have to weigh the potential benefits of this therapy against its possible future side effects.

LIVER EFFECTS

Early studies linking high doses of testosterone with liver cancer in men caused alarm, and many physicians still cling to the idea that testosterone is a liver enemy. But subsequent studies of women have found no serious liver side effects, no changes in liver function and no harmful effect on liver enzymes when physiological doses of testosterone were given.

BREAST AND UTERINE CANCER CONCERNS

Whenever a hormone therapy is suggested, we are worried about its effect on our risk of breast and uterine cancer. In the past, high doses of testosterone were used to treat breast cancer. It didn't help, but it didn't hurt either. When testosterone is added to estrogen it will not prevent buildup of the uterine lining caused by the estrogen; thus it will not protect against uterine cancer. For that reason, if a woman has her uterus and takes estrogen, she must still take a progestin, even if she takes testosterone.

WHO SHOULD CONSIDER TAKING TESTOSTERONE?

In order to determine this, we need to look at our symptoms, our age and our hormonal status.

SYMPTOMS OF ANDROGEN DEFICIENCY

If you experience a diminished sense of well-being in addition to one or more of the following symptoms, you should have your blood levels of free testosterone checked:

- Significant loss of libido that is global (no one or no thing turns you on)

- Loss of ability to become aroused no matter what you or your partner do
- Notable decrease in sensitivity in the nipples and or clitoris
- Loss of ability to have orgasm, or severe diminishment in the quality of orgasm
- Loss of pubic hair

TIMING IT RIGHT

There are certain periods in our lives when androgen deficiency can develop.

BEFORE PERIMENOPAUSE

Consider androgen replacement if you have severe symptoms of androgen deficiency and/or you are taking a medication that significantly lowers free testosterone levels, such as birth control pills, antidepressants, anti-anxiety medications or blood-pressure-lowering medications (for a complete—and very long—list, see Chapter 7). But consider supplementing only if your free testosterone level is indeed low. Note: There are practically no studies that examine the use of testosterone in women in this age group. Also note that women of reproductive age who have normal testosterone levels won't benefit from adding extra testosterone. This is not a magic bullet!

DURING PERIMENOPAUSE

Testosterone supplementation may help if you develop symptoms of androgen deficiency, especially with other perimenopausal signs of hormone loss.

DURING MENOPAUSE

If you have signs of androgen deficiency or if you do not achieve satisfactory relief of your menopausal symptoms with estrogen replacement alone, consider adding male hormone. Also talk to your

VAGINAL DRYNESS AND PAIN

Jane was referred to me by her rheumatologist, who treated her for mild rheumatoid arthritis. She is a 43-year-old data processer who has been married for 10 years. She used birth control pills until the age of 37 and quit taking them when her husband had a vasectomy. Her cycles were irregular, and she had major mood swings until a year ago, when her periods stopped. Since then, she has had mild hot flashes, but her moodiness has improved. Jane's chief complaint was extreme vaginal dryness and pain with intercourse. She had tried lubricants and moisturizers, but still felt that she was being torn every time she and her husband attempt penetration. They stopped trying, and she wondered if she cared.

Jane's mother died of pancreatic cancer at the age of 62, and her sister was diagnosed with breast cancer at age 39. So Jane had decided that she would "do" menopause without estrogen. She exercises, eats right and takes calcium and vitamins. Her cholesterol and lipid profiles are fine. So far, her mammograms have been normal.

When I examined Jane, I found that she had severe genital atrophy. The labia were thin, and insertion of even a small speculum was painful and difficult. Her vaginal walls were pale, dry and smooth. I didn't have to do blood tests to see how very hormone-deficient she was. We performed a bone density scan, which showed that Jane had already lost about 20 percent of her ideal bone mass from age 30. Her blood tests confirmed that she was menopausal. Her total testosterone was less than 10 nanograms/per deciliter(normal is 20 to 80 nanograms/dl), and her free testosterone was negligible. Because Jane's only menopausal complaint was her severe vaginal dryness and atrophy (which could have been compounded by her autoimmune disease), we decided to attack with local therapy.

She started with estrogen cream, which she would insert daily to build up the vaginal walls. I also gave her a set of expanding dilators to insert as the area felt more comfortable and stretchable. She began using the Estring vaginal ring as soon as she was able to insert it. Estring gives out only two milligrams of estradiol over three months and will probably have an insignificant effect on her estrogen blood levels. I also prescribed 2-percent testosterone propionate ointment to be used on the clitoris and vulva. Finally, she started taking Evista, a selective estrogen that will bind to the receptors in her bone and help prevent osteoporosis without activating estrogen receptors in her breasts or uterus.

Four months later, Jane is able (with lots of lubrication) to have intercourse. She still feels tight, but the more she practices, the better it gets. She found the testosterone ointment to be too "gunky," and she started using 0.5-milligram methyltestosterone troches, which she puts under her tongue daily to raise her male hormone levels. Since the hurt went away, she looks forward to having sex.

doctor about taking testosterone if you already have osteoporosis or are at high risk of developing this disease.

AFTER SURGICAL, RADIATION OR CHEMOTHERAPEUTIC DESTRUCTION OF THE OVARIES

This may be the strongest indication for taking testosterone, in addition to estrogen.

WHO SHOULD *NOT* BE TAKING TESTOSTERONE?

Because of the possible side effects listed above, and the complete lack of long-term studies on male hormone supplementation in women, we all should play it very safe. I currently recommend that you not take testosterone in the following situations unless you and your doctor feel that the benefits overwhelm the possible risks:

PREGNANCY

This is the most clear-cut contraindication to the use of testosterone. Exposing a pregnant woman to male hormone will cause virilization of the developing fetus—a disaster no matter what the sex of the baby. Unless you are using foolproof birth control and can't conceivably conceive, you should steer clear of male hormones.

CHRONIC DISEASES

Because we are not sure about testosterone's effect on heart disease in women, it might be unwise to add this hormone if you are already at very high risk for developing cardiovascular disease (in other words, if you have diabetes, hypertension, uncontrolled high cholesterol levels or perhaps a very strong family history of heart disease). Because smoking, obesity and sedentary lifestyle are also heart offenders, it would be wise to stop or change these cardiac insults if you want to jump-start your sex life with testosterone.

LIVER DISEASE

Although it takes very high doses of testosterone to damage the liver, if you start out with a damaged liver, testosterone may be the straw that breaks the liver's back.

ANDROGEN EXCESS DISORDERS

If you have polycystic ovary syndrome or another condition that causes overproduction of male hormone, testosterone is unnecessary. Moreover, because of the risk of coronary artery disease linked with these conditions, extra testosterone could add insult to injury.

ACNE AND MALE PATTERN BALDING

Testosterone may make both of these conditions worse.

PREVIOUS BREAST CANCER

Large doses of testosterone given to women who have had breast cancer did not increase recurrence rates. However, there is concern about giving even physiological doses of natural testosterone (as opposed to the synthetic kind) to women with current or past breast cancer. Natural testosterone can be converted to estrogens by the body. This concern may not be warranted, and more and more studies are showing that women who have had breast cancer and who take estrogen replacement do not risk an increase in recurrence, metastases or mortality. But the testosterone-becoming-estrogen issue can be partially bypassed by using synthetic testosterone (usually methyltestosterone; see below). I have many patients who are very libido-deprived after breast cancer chemotherapy. They have had to cope with the trauma of diagnosis, surgery and severe menopausal symptoms, and they are not willing to forgo the pleasures of sex. They want to take androgens and often are also willing to take estrogen. After discussion of all the pros and cons, I prescribe one or both.

TESTS YOU NEED BEFORE TAKING TESTOSTERONE

Obviously, we have to make sure that your "I'm not in the mood . . ." feeling is not due to a medical condition, and conversely that you do not have a medical condition that might prevent you from taking testosterone. These are the tests I recommend:

- **Thyroid function** (thyroid stimulating hormone, or TSH, test) to screen for thyroid abnormalities
- **Complete blood count** to rule out anemia
- **Prolactin level measurement** to rule out pituitary tumors
- **Liver function tests** to make sure your liver is healthy
- **Cholesterol and lipid profile** to get a baseline for future comparison, in the event that you take testosterone, and to ensure that levels are not abnormal
- **Free testosterone level test.** This is our most important gauge of testosterone deficiency and the need for supplementation.
- **DHEAS level measurement.** If your DHEAS level is low, your testosterone woes may be due to lack of adrenal production, and adding DHEA supplementation (see below) may be the way to go.
- **FSH level measurement.** It will be elevated if you are menopausal or close to menopause.

PILLS, PATCHES, CREAMS OR SHOTS: HOW SHOULD WE TAKE TESTOSTERONE?

There is no one testosterone. This appellation really applies generically to the hormone that is circulating in our body (and even then, we distinguish between that which is bound and that which is free). When natural testosterone is given orally, its half-life is just 10 to 20 minutes. It is quickly broken down in the digestive tract. This breakdown can be diminished by the process of micronization—chopping testosterone into thousands of granules—or by suspending it in an oil solution. What some pharmaceutical companies have done to ensure a slower, steadier absorption is to synthesize a methylated form, to prevent breakdown.

Once natural testosterone gets into our body, what is not broken down will be converted to an estrogen. This does not happen with the synthetic methyltestosterone, so we get a bigger testosterone bang for the pill. The metabolism of testosterone and much of its conversion to estrogen occurs in the liver. Whenever we swallow a pill or capsule, the medication must first travel to our liver before it gets into the bloodstream. This is called "first bypass." If the hormone is absorbed directly into the bloodstream through the skin or the mucous membranes of the vagina or mouth, or is given as an injection, it will not go directly to the liver and avoids first bypass. We should also remember that testosterone exerts its effect on our lipid profile in the liver. So it stands to reason that when that organ is initially skipped, there is much less chance of adverse cholesterol effects.

So we have a choice: natural testosterone versus synthetic methyltestosterone. To add to our dilemma, either of these can be administered through capsules, tablets, ointments, gels, patches or troches (lozenges placed under the tongue).

The only testosterone made by a pharmaceutical company that is currently available in the United States, listed in the *Physicians' Desk Reference* and suitable for testosterone replacement purposes in women is methyltestosterone. Its sole approved use is "for treatment of moderate to severe vasomotor symptoms associated with the menopause in patients not improved by estrogen alone." Moreover, it is manufactured only with esterified estrogen, not on its own. Sold under the brand name Estratest by Solvay Pharmaceuticals, it comes

in two strengths: The higher dose contains 1.25 milligrams of esterified estrogen and 2.5 milligrams methyltestosterone, and the lower
dose, Estratest H.S. (this stands for half strength—not a particularly winning marketing term), contains 0.625 milligrams of esterified estrogen and 1.25 milligrams methyltestosterone. That doesn't
give us a lot of options if we are going to limit our male hormone
supplementation to brand names.

This is where formulating, or "compounding," pharmacies may
become our friend. They are the ones that can take natural or synthetic testosterone and concoct the capsules, creams, gels, ointments
and lozenges mentioned earlier. They will not, however, do this without a prescription from a doctor. Testosterone is a controlled
substance.

When all our systems are on "go" and we are making our own
testosterone in our ovaries and adrenal glands, we produce about 1.25
milligrams per day. This gives us total serum levels that range from
12 to 90 nanograms per deciliter, which is what we want to achieve
with testosterone replacement. Even Estratest H.S. may be too
strong, so what I suggest my patients do, especially if they develop
acne or hirsutism (or if I'm unhappy with their cholesterol profile),
is take Estratest H.S. every other day and supply their dose of estrogen
on the no-testosterone days with Estratab (Solvay's form of esterified estrogen). I practically never prescribe the higher-dose
Estratest.

If possible, I like to avoid the liver (I don't eat liver either) and in
order to prevent first bypass, I frequently prescribe methyltestosterone
troches which are placed under the tongue so that the hormone is
absorbed directly into the bloodstream. There is a testosterone patch
created for men, made by Smithkline Beecham, but it is too strong
for us and I'm still awaiting data on its use in women (I understand
that a patch for women is currently being tested). I generally do not

prescribe long-acting injections, because they overdose initially and underdose as the shot begins to wear off.

So what happened to the creams, gels and ointments? After I talked on the *Oprah Winfrey Show* about the use of testosterone propionate ointment on the external genitalia, there was a general consensus that every woman in America should greet her gynecologist with, "Show me the cream!" This local testosterone application in an area of extreme testosterone receptorship sounds too good to be true. On occasion, the results are amazing: The clitoris and surrounding tissue respond with a healthy thickening and increased sensitivity. Moreover, a small amount of the testosterone gets absorbed and has a system-wide effect. The absorption can be variable and, in my experience, one-fourth of a teaspoon of 1-percent to 2-percent testosterone ointment, used no more than once a day, will not cause nonphysiological testosterone levels or masculinization. After two months, when the local testosterone receptors have been given a boost, I generally have my patients apply the ointment just three times weekly.

Ointment sits on the tissues and is poorly absorbed, so it does its "thing" locally. Gels and creams are absorbed far more rapidly and therefore should be used in a much lower dose—just 0.2 percent of a rapidly absorbing organogel has a physiological effect. To obfuscate the issue, natural testosterone can be mixed into a cream or gel that will be broken down more quickly once absorbed into the body. Or testosterone can be synthetically bonded to propionate, a chemical that reduces metabolism. This too can be mixed with a cream or ointment. Creams and gels can be absorbed through the skin at other sites on our body and can be a medium for general use.

The following are some of the testosterone preparations that can be prescribed:

TYPES OF TESTOSTERONE

MANUFACTURED BY PHARMACEUTICAL COMPANIES

TABLETS

Estratest
    Esterified estrogens   1.25 mg
    Methyltestosterone   2.5 mg
Estratest H.S.
    Esterified estrogens   0.625 mg
    Methyltestosterone   1.25 mg

PATCHES (doses currently used for men)

Androderm 2.5 (testosterone)   12.2 mg; releases 2.5 mg/day

Androderm 5   24.3 mg; releases 5 mg/day

INJECTIONS

Testosterone cypionate   50 mg/dl

Testosterone enenthate   90 mg/ml

PREPARED BY COMPOUNDING PHARMACIES

CAPSULES

Micronized testosterone in oil   0.25 mg and higher

Methyltestosterone   0.5 mg and higher

TROCHES (lozenges) or tablets, placed under the tongue

Methyltestosterone   0.2 mg and higher

Testosterone   0.5 mg and higher

DROPS, placed under the tongue

Testosterone   0.5 mg/0.2 ml

CREAMS

Testosterone proprionate   0.25% and higher

Testosterone	0.25% and higher

OINTMENT (petroleum based)	
Testosterone proprionate	1 to 2%

GEL Organogel, a lipid and water gel that allows increased absorption	
Testosterone	0.1 to 1.5%

This is a huge "compounded" list. I have my own favorites when I prescribe testosterone for my patients: the methyltestosterone troques for systemic supplementation and either testosterone proprionate ointment or testosterone organogel for local therapy. To find a local compounding pharmacy that will fill your physician's prescription, call the International Association of Compounding Pharmacies at 1-800-927-4227.

THE TESTOSTERONE TRACKING SYSTEM

When I give estrogen, I know what's going in and what it will do. I have myriad studies telling me that 0.625 milligrams of Premarin or conjugated estrogen is equivalent to 1 milligram of estradiol, which equals 0.5 milligrams in a patch. I even know what blood levels to expect if I give estrogen in a vaginal cream or ring. But when it comes to testosterone, there are no tables, no equivalencies and no data on blood levels. Moreover, no one has figured out how long it is "safe" to use it. What we do know is that if we're in a state of testosterone deficiency, it is not going to go away on its own. Here is what I do to monitor my patients:

- I have them come back to the office three to six months after starting therapy so that I can discuss any positive (or negative) effects they have experienced.

- I tell them to watch for symptoms such as acne, hirsutism and male pattern hair loss and notify me if these occur. (These symptoms seldom occur before the first follow-up visit.)
- When they return, I retest their cholesterol profile (total, HDL, LDL, triglycerides) and if they were taking natural testosterone in any form, I might retest their free testosterone level. (It's useless, as you can understand by now, to test free testosterone if they are taking methyltestosterone.)
- Thereafter, at their yearly checkup, I test their cholesterol, liver function and whatever needs to be checked for their general health.

So that's it, folks. We're still searching for the right way, the right dose and the right duration. Until we know more, we have to use clinical success and laboratory tests as our guide.

DHEA: THE OTHER MALE HORMONE

When it comes to knowledge about testosterone and its supplementation in women, we are in the Middle Ages. When it comes to another male hormone, DHEA, we're in the Dark Ages. DHEA's purported fountain-of-youth qualities (or at least those that produce a puddle of diminished aging) have been tested almost exclusively on rats and men. Philosophically, we may not want to attach ourselves to either research category, but there are more pragmatic reasons for a separation. Rats barely produce their own DHEA, so when we supply them with this hormone and proudly point to the fact that the treated rats have less diabetes, obesity, heart disease and cancer, live longer, and even learn better, we are drawing conclusions that may have no validity in DHEA-producing humans.

The researchers have acknowledged this and passed on to a higher, but gender-specific species—man. Men, however, have higher levels of DHEA than women. These levels may be significant in protecting their health, possibly because they don't have estrogen to do it. Men with low levels of DHEA are more likely than those whose natural levels are higher to have heart attacks and prostate cancer. If men are given huge amounts of DHEA (1,600 milligrams), their lipid profiles improve, they become more insulin-sensitive and their male hormones are hardly affected.

None of this seems to apply to women. There is no correlation between our basic DHEA levels and coronary vascular disease, nor has one been found for breast cancer. Giving 1,600 milligrams of DHEA to women causes disastrous changes in their lipid profiles and could actually increase their risk of heart attack. The only survey in which we seem to share a benefit is one that showed that both men and women who developed Alzheimer's had lower DHEA levels than those who did not.

Having rendered this ratty masculine introduction, let me go on to tell you what we do know about DHEA in women. At their peak, our adrenal glands are the busiest hormone-producing organs in our bodies. They make DHEA, which is quickly converted to DHEAS (DHEA-sulfate). This conversion is there to protect our DHEA stores; otherwise, we would run short. When allowed to roam free, DHEA has only a 25-minute half-life (the period of time after which one-half of it will be broken down and disappear). DHEAS, however, has a 10-hour half-life. We have 300 to 500 times more DHEAS than its DHEA precursor, and the former is the most abundant hormone in our body. This constitutes a huge pool of available prohormone, which bathes all of our systems and can be converted to androstendione, testosterone, dehydrotestosterone or even estrogen (see Chapter 3). Some of this change from prohormone to hormone takes place in our adrenals and ovaries, but mostly it occurs in cells and tissues in the rest of our body. Seventy percent of all estrogen and androgen is synthesized from DHEAS before menopause, and close to 100 percent after. We peak in our DHEAS production in our late twenties, and this level falls by 50 percent in our forties. The subsequent decline of DHEAS is accelerated by menopause, and we end up losing 70 to 95 percent as we continue to age. This is our adrenopause. The question we need to ask is whether adrenopause contributes to changes in our metabolism and the development of diabetes, obesity, cardiovascular disease, cancer and lack of immune response in our later years. Or, are these later years simply causing our adrenals to slow down or come to a standstill? More simply, do our adrenals age because we do, or do we age because our adrenals have failed us? In the face of this monumental question, it may seem insignificant to ask, does adrenopause cause libido-pause?

SO WHAT CAN DHEA SUPPLEMENTATION DO FOR US?

As expected, if we take DHEA orally, it will go through our liver, where, within one to two hours, it undergoes bioconversion to testosterone. A 100-milligram tablet causes a fourfold increase in this androgen; a 50-milligram tablet causes a twofold increase, and the elevation continues for 12 hours. These numbers were obtained from studies performed on very small groups of postmenopausal women, and the duration of these studies ranged from just a few weeks to one year. A two- to fourfold increase in testosterone sounds like a lot, but the levels were still lower than those present in most premenopausal women. It doesn't matter—the numbers scared most researchers, who then concluded that this might not be the thing to do to women. There were some mild lipid changes in about half of the studies using 100 to 500 milligrams of DHEA. There was a decrease in cholesterol, HDL, LDL and triglycerides. So here, too, the experts correctly stated that the long-term cardiovascular effect of DHEA supplementation, even in low doses of 50 milligrams or less, is unknown (what is known is that we will need decades, not weeks, of study to draw any conclusions).

Since we don't have information on long-term side effects, what about short-term beneficial effects? DHEA supplementation does not seem to help women respond to insulin, lose body fat or lose weight. It may help us get better REM sleep and improve our sense of well-being (this last statement has been brought to you by a study on just 17 women followed for fewer than six months!). DHEA may also help older individuals (which, of course, includes women) respond to vaccines with better antibody production. Just three weeks of DHEA therapy was shown to activate natural killer cells that are important in preventing growth of cancer cells. Two hundred milligrams of DHEA improves symptoms in many women with lupus. That's it for the studies, and none of them has shown that DHEA supplementation improved libido (although in all fairness, the researchers didn't always ask whether it did).

SHOULD I USE DHEA AS MY MALE HORMONE SUPPLEMENT IF I NEED ONE?

Since I have no documentation of libido improvement, I cannot currently recommend DHEA as a male hormone booster that will enhance our sexual function. I suspect that because it does raise our total and free testosterone levels, it may, in the future, be found to have some sexual value. Having said this, I have to admit that I recommend it to my patients who complain of diminished libido together with low energy and poor sense of well-being if their blood levels of DHEAS are low. I usually prescribe 25 milligrams and never more than 50 milligrams a day. I also monitor their lipids and testosterone levels.

"Prescribe" is a misnomer—DHEA is not currently regulated as a pharmaceutical and can be bought without a prescription as a vitamin supplement. The resulting production and marketing chaos means that quantity and quality control are not guaranteed. We don't know exactly how much or what is in the pill. Most DHEA tablets are plain, crystalline DHEA, and when they are ingested, they are subject to first bypass in the liver, with a high rate of conversion to testosterone. This might give us an androgen advantage, but if we are taking the pill for its supposed DHEA benefits, we're in the wrong hormone park and throwing out the DHEA at the beginning of the game.

Micronization of the DHEA (chopping it into thousands of minuscule pieces) and suspension in oil will prevent some of this liver breakdown. The oil base encourages direct absorption of the active DHEA into our lymph system, so we get more bang for the dose. This form of micronized DHEA is made by compounding pharmacies and usually requires a prescription. As with testosterone, DHEA can also be put in a cream. This decreases first bypass in the liver and allows the peripheral cells to do most of the conversion to androgen and estrogen. A Canadian researcher is testing this and feels that ultimately, it may allow us to safely correct deficiencies of our sex hormones on a cellular basis.

Our unproven so-called fountain of youth may yet become a dew of better and longer life. In the process, perhaps we'll discover that it also helps us feel sexy.

CHAPTER THIRTEEN

MORE THAN HORMONES:

Alternatives and Adjuncts

I N OUR FRENZIED SEARCH for a modern libido potion, we may forget that there is a 5,000-year-old tradition of pursuing better sex through chemistry—with foods, herbs and natural drugs.

What parent wouldn't be disturbed to have her daughter taken out on a date and fed *oysters?* The thought, of course, is that the conniving male is giving this pure, unsuspecting young woman an aphrodisiac that will undermine her judgment and get her to acquiesce to sex. Our sexual expectations of seafood stem from the mythological tradition of Aphrodite, the Greek goddess of sexual love and beauty. She came from the sea and was thought to have imbued her essence into oysters (which would lead us to assume that scallops, shrimp and even the lowly flounder also possess aphrodisiac qualities). Naturally, this is based on no science whatsoever. The only science is that raw shellfish can give us hepatitis A and that coldwater fish contains Omega-3 fatty acids, which protect our heart. But a healthy heart leads to good sex, so perhaps we should go for it . . .

Other so-called aphrodisiacs earned their purported power because they grow in the shape of a phallus. *Rhinocerous horn* obviously fits the mold. There is no proof that it works, but because of a near-religious belief in the powers of a powder made from the exotic substance, an amazing animal has been hunted almost to the point of extinction.

A less ecologically harmful product is *ginseng*, and there has been some research into its powers—in mice and men. (The word *ginseng* means "man root," so why should researchers bother to check its effect in women?) In Korea, researchers compared a group of men taking ginseng to those given a placebo. The ginseng group felt that the root did not change their frequency of intercourse or morning erections, but the rigidity and girth of their penises improved, and the men reported that their libido was significantly higher. This may partially be due to the fact that ginseng can have a mild stimulant action like coffee.

Other studies in humans have not been quite as impressive, so researchers decided to bring in the rats. They observed that male rats treated with ginseng had sex more frequently, but they also ejaculated earlier (not necessarily a good thing). These copulating rats also seemed to gain protection against heat stress, physical stress and electroshock. (The poor rodents must have associated sex with torture!)

And speaking of torture, some aphrodisiacs do just that. *Spanish fly* is made from dried beetle remains. (In the United States, perhaps we could use the more ubiquitous cockroach.) When the insect byproduct is excreted in urine, it irritates the urogenital tract, causing blood to rush to the rescue and engorge the genitals. This can lead to bladder infections, scarring of the urethra and death—a high price to pay for sexual improvement.

Irritation is associated with other aphrodisiacs as well. This might explain why *chilies, curries and other spicy foods* that stimulate our gastric acids and our nervous system are rumored to have potency powers. But any power they have is probably connected to the fact that they cause reactions similar to those that occur during sex: a faster heartbeat and sweating. Or perhaps their power lies in the fact that if we believe something is going to be a sexual stimulant, the belief itself is stimulating.

Such is the case with *pollen, royal jelly and honey*, all of which come from the honeybee. These are popular as general energy-boosters and sex-enhancers, especially among the French. I found no reliable data on this.

But let's not discount sweets altogether. *Chocolate*, as anyone who has had PMS knows, stimulates pleasure (by raising serotonin levels in the brain) and gives us that warm, happy feeling of first love. It is not an aphrodisiac, but it is a safe, albeit fattening, way to achieve satisfaction.

HERBS

Ginseng may be our best-known potency herb, but others have been studied and even given a degree of scientific blessing.

YOHIMBINE

This substance taken from the bark of the African Yohimbe tree has been used for centuries in Africa and West India and is thought to stimulate the nervous-system activity that promotes erection. It may also improve mood and decrease anxiety. When it was given to men with erectile difficulties, some studies showed an impressive improvement, but others questioned these results. And none of them looked at the effects in women.

Yohimbine has been found to counteract some of the erectile difficulties in men taking SSRI antidepressants (see Chapter 5). Extracts from the Yohimbe tree can be purchased in health food stores in both capsule and tincture forms. Yohimbine hydrochloride, the most active chemical compound in Yohimbe bark, is available by prescription under the brand names Yocon, Yohimex, Aphrodyne and

Erex (marketing strategies never cease to amaze me). Both the over-the-counter and prescription versions of this substance should be taken carefully and under a physician's supervision. High doses can elevate blood pressure and heart rate and cause sweating, nausea and vomiting. These warnings pertain to men; we don't yet have data to allow us to give warnings to women. The *Physicians' Desk Reference* says of yohimbine hydrochloride, "this drug is not proposed for use in females."

BLACK COHOSH
This herb is found in the woodlands of eastern North America and has been used as a menopause remedy in Germany for decades. Exten-sive European studies show standardized extracts of its root (sold in health food stores under the brand name Remifemin) can successfully treat several menopausal symptoms, including hot flashes, sleep dis-turbances and vaginal dryness. When all these are improved, our abil-ity to have sex and achieve satisfaction may improve as well.

SAW PALMETTO
This substance, sold in health food stores, comes from a shrub that grows along the Atlantic coast and is purported to promote sexual potency by strengthening the reproductive system. Historically, a tea made from the shrub's berries was popular with Native Americans. Unfortunately, what little research there has been into saw palmetto's powers has focused on its use in the treatment of prostate disease. No one has looked at its effect on women.

OTHER HERBS
Additional herbs that have been included in a list of love potions with no scientific demonstration of their effectiveness are licorice, sarsaparilla, myrtle, Chinese tea tree (or Ti-tree), kava kava, echina-cea and damiana. Dong quai, a plant estrogen, is often included in

herbal formulations for women. Some women report that it helps ease PMS and menopausal symptoms and, as such, may make them feel more "in the mood," but there is no evidence that it has any special aphrodisiac properties.

PROSEXUAL MEDICATIONS

We know that drugs are among our chief sex saboteurs, but there is also the possibility that we can achieve better sex through medicine with the following:

VIAGRA

This very successful new "up" drug for the treatment of erectile disorders in men could eventually help out women as well. (For exhaustive details, see Chapter 11.) As usual, the medication was invented for and tested only in men, but to their gender-equating credit (both emotional and financial), Pfizer, the drug's manufacturer, is conducting European trials of Viagra in women. We would expect it to improve arousal by increasing blood flow to the genitals, lubrication and clitoral response, and indeed, a spokesperson for the company has verified this does occur and may increase responsiveness to sexual stimulation in some women. Viagra has not been shown to have an effect on women's libido, nor is there a documented improvement in their orgasmic response. (The researchers understandably point out that because orgasm in women is so multifactorial, verification of improvement is hard to come by.) In the future Viagra may be important to women who develop vaginal atrophy and who cannot, or choose not, to use hormone therapy.

We may also be the recipients of fallout from investigations on other impotence drugs currently being tested in men. These include phentolamine (Vasomax), which dilates blood vessels; apomorphine (Spontane), which acts on the central nervous system; and prostaglandin creams, which stimulate blood flow when applied to the surface of the genitals.

L-DOPA (LARADOPA)

This precursor of dopamine is used to treat Parkinson's disease, and it has been found that some male patients taking it exhibit a heightened interest in sex and improved sexual function. Because L-Dopa inhibits the release of prolactin and promotes production of dopamine, it is chemically suited to be a libido booster. However, all but one of the studies noting its sexual effects have been of patients with Parkinson's disease, and the sole study done specifically on those with erectile dysfunction included no women. Furthermore, its potential side effects, which include nausea, vomiting, headache and cardiac irregularities, are a serious turn-off.

BROMOCRIPTINE (PARLODEL)

This drug is given to reduce prolactin levels in people with certain tumors of the pituitary gland. Any condition that causes prolactin levels to rise can stop our periods, cause infertility and diminish our production of male hormone. When a man seeks medical therapy for erectile dysfunction, one of the tests that is routinely performed is a check of his blood prolactin level. Women with menstrual irregularity or secretion of fluid from their breasts should be given the same test and, if their levels are high, the same drug. Thankfully, few of us can blame our diminished libido on a brain tumor.

DEPRENYL (ELDEPRYL)

This prescription medication, used to treat Parkinson's disease, inhibits MAO B, an enzyme in the brain that breaks down neurotransmitters such as dopamine and serotonin. Dopamine has been shown to improve libido, while serotonin may have the opposite effect. The question is, which of these chemicals will emerge as the winner? And will the overall effect be one of improved libido? Because this medication affects neurotransmitters, it should not be used with SSRI antidepressants or other drugs that affect neurotransmitter levels without consultation with a psychopharmacologist.

ANTIDEPRESSANTS

We've already discussed trazadone (Desyrel) and buproprion (Wellbutrin) as alternatives to mood-boosting medications that impair sexual function. Because these may actually be prosexual drugs, their potential for use by nondepressed individuals certainly warrants research and consideration.

PHEROMONES AND SCENT

Just as we would like aphrodisiacs to heighten our sexual response, we would like to find a smell—preferably one we could bottle and sell—to do the same. But are pheromones the aroma of love? Will a "little dab do us"? There is no question that part of what attracts one animal to another is scent, and most mammals detect the odor of attraction, called pheromones, through the vomeronasal organ (VNO) in the nose. This scent may not be perceptible to humans in the same way that other smells are. There is an ongoing debate as to whether we even have a VNO, much less know how to use it. What we do know is that chemicals found in sweat and other secretions can affect the body functions of women who live or work together. In one study of 135 women, cloth pads placed under the arms of a group of women living in one dormitory were rubbed under the noses of a second group living in a different dorm. Gradually, the periods of the women in the second group became synchronized with those of the women in the first.

What does all this mean as far as sexual desire goes? Are those of us who secrete more pheromones perceived as sexier? Is our society's addiction to perfumes, deodorants, antiperspirants and all of the other products that mask our natural scent inhibiting our attractiveness? Women's sense of smell is naturally more acute than men's, so are pheromones—if they exist—more important for luring us to a specific man than vice versa? Manufacturers hoping to capitalize on this query have used the word "pheromone" in their product's name. They claim to have isolated substances with pheromones' chemical properties, among them byproducts of DHEA. Whether this is brilliant science or just a brilliant marketing gimmick is up for grabs. We don't know if the nose knows.

Rather than trying to re-create glandular substances and body secretions, researchers at the Smell and Taste Treatment and Research Foundation in Chicago took a more palatable approach. After testing the effects of a variety of odors, they found that a combination of black licorice candy, cucumber, baby powder, lavender and pumpkin pie caused the greatest increase in female sexual arousal. Black licorice plus cucumber was the most arousing scent; cherry was the most inhibiting. In support of the pheromone theory, the researchers found that men's cologne actually reduced arousal levels. So much for all those wonderful, sexy ads showing men with great bodies anointing themselves and then attracting gorgeous models. I'll miss them—the men, that is.

In my quest for sex-enhancing alternatives and adjuncts, I visited several health food stores and scanned the shelves. I also browsed the Internet. I was astounded by the number of products and their wonderfully descriptive names (Eros, Herbal Passion, Lover's Tea, Intima for Women, Vigorex). But I was dismayed by the fact that the subtle inferences and outright claims of the products' sexual powers were not substantiated, at least not to my satisfaction. I have contemplated trying many of these products in order to be a sacrificial guinea pig on behalf of this book, but as a physician, I cannot accept or disseminate personal anecdotal experiences as proof of a product's efficacy. Nor should you. Now on to adjuncts that *have* been shown to improve sex . . .

LUBRICANTS AND MOISTURIZERS

Unwanted friction causes unwanted wear, tear and pain. Mechanical engineers know this, which is why they invented motor oil. When we don't have essential vaginal lubrication during arousal, penetration is inevitably unpleasurable, if not downright painful. Vaginal dryness may be caused by a decline in estrogen or be a side effect of medication. If that sandpaper feeling is hormone-related, total-body estrogen replacement with pills or patches, and/or locally applied estrogen creams or vaginal rings, is the most effective way to improve our natural secretions.

But many women can't or won't use hormones, and that shouldn't sentence them to a lifetime of uncomfortable sex. They can moisturize their vaginal and vulvar tissue and use lubricants to glide through sex. Moisturizers such as Gyne-Moistrin, Replens and Vagisil need to be used regularly (sometimes every day, sometimes every few days) in order to work. They are not for dryness emergencies only. Lubricants are; they should be applied to the labia, clitoris or vagina, or to a partner's penis during foreplay. (Don't be afraid to reapply just before or during penetration.) There are various brands available; these include Astroglide, K-Y Lotion, Lubrin, Moist Again and Touch. Vaseline is not a good lubricant; it can cake or dry and weakens condoms. Also resist the urge to use perfumed lotions or oils, which can cause vaginal and penile irritation.

LIFESTYLE CHANGES

This is my public service announcement. If you want better sex, take care of your health. Doing so takes time, effort and commitment and may be our most arduous libido enhancer, but it's cheaper than a lifetime supply of Viagra and well worth it. Let's go through the basics:

EXERCISE

Regular physical activity raises endorphins (our internal feel-good hormones), boosts energy, increases stamina, tones muscles, strengthens bones, keeps our weight down and improves our body image. I probably should not have to say more, but I will. A study at the University of Washington showed that an intense 20-minute workout on an exercise bike had an effect on subsequent arousal. When compared to women who didn't exercise, those who had just worked out experienced a greater increase in blood flow to the vagina in response to an erotic film. This means that exercising with your partner could be a before-foreplay arousal enhancer. A word of caution: Excessive exercise, especially in conjunction with weight loss, can diminish our ovarian function and result in lowered estrogen, progesterone and testosterone levels, all of which can hamper sexual desire, function and pleasure. The same goes for your partner: If he starts working out for several hours a day or trains for a marathon, both his testosterone level and his erection may dwindle. And if his chosen form of exercise is intense or prolonged bicycling, that ridiculous little seat may press on vital arteries in the penis and his exercise challenge can evolve into an erection challenge. Women cyclists are not immune: They may experience trauma to the vulva and develop clitoral numbness and orgasmic dysfunction.

Not all exercise is created equal, and some has special benefits, toning and strengthening the muscles that contract during sex. Kegel exercises involve isolating and repeatedly contracting the muscles that allow us to squeeze our vagina. The best way to find these muscles is to put your finger in your vagina and squeeze. After isolating the muscles that "close down" on your finger, remove it and contract these muscles for 10 seconds, then relax for 10 seconds. This should be repeated 15 to 25 times, and ideally the entire workout should be done three times a day. It is certainly not painful and will be sexually gainful.

DIET

We all know what we should eat to promote good health and prevent obesity. The timing and size of our meals may also be a factor in the timing and pleasure of sex. Heavy meals diminish arousal by elevating serotonin levels, and too much alcohol is a sexual saboteur.

VITAMINS AND MINERALS

Once more, the evidence is anecdotal. There are those who advocate the use of B vitamins to enhance energy and blood flow and antioxidants to help keep blood vessels healthy, ensuring a steady supply of blood to the genitals. The amino acid proponents claim that these building blocks of all our proteins are necessary for healthy neurotransmitter function and thus improve erection and stimulation.

Practically every vitamin and mineral has been touted as an aid to our sexuality and libido, but the paucity of evidence precludes my prostrating myself before this nutrient-power proclamation. I do recommend that my patients take a multivitamin containing 400 micrograms of folic acid, as well as 400 international units of vitamin E and 500 to 1,000 milligrams of vitamin C for general health benefits. I also tell them to take 1,200 to 1,500 milligrams of calcium (or the equivalent in foods). Eighty percent of us do not get enough calcium for our bones, and although we rarely associate sexual function with

bone density, women with severe osteoporosis and compression fractures of their spine are in no position—literally—to avail themselves
of the pleasures of sexual intercourse.

While we acknowledge that most of us are calcium deficient, we
pay less attention to another mineral, zinc. In men, zinc has been
shown to be essential for prostate gland function and to help in the
production of sperm. It is also involved in the synthesis of dehydrotestosterone, the final, active form of male hormone in both men and
women. Is there a nationwide epidemic of zinc deficiency, and do we
need extra zinc to enhance sex? Once more the evidence is deficient.
But if you're looking for zinc-induced zest, you might find it in oysters,
which are high in this mineral. So perhaps they do have some aphrodisiac qualities after all . . .

SMOKING

Hollywood has long used the lighting of a cigarette to signal post-sex
satisfaction. But the truth is that this seemingly sexy cigarette will
diminish sexual proclivity and prowess by damaging blood vessels
throughout the body, including those that are necessary for arousal.
No one—not even the tobacco companies—has suggested that any
of the 4,000 chemicals that enter our body through cigarette smoke
has aphrodisiac qualities. Furthermore, the consequences of smoking,
such as heart attack, stroke, lung cancer, emphysema and of course
death, will physically prevent us or our partners from engaging in sex.

On an up note, it has been found that women ages 52 to 62 who
stop smoking experience an increase in sexual frequency. A new drug,
marketed under the name Zyban, is currently being prescribed to help
us quit and has the added benefit of preventing the appetite changes
and weight gain that so many would-be nonsmokers fear. This drug
is actually buproprion, better known as Wellbutrin, an antidepressant
whose sex-enhancing properties were already discussed. So while
we're kicking the habit, we may also be kicking up our libido.

CHAPTER FOURTEEN

CAN WE TALK?

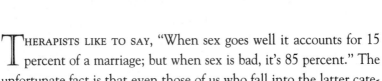

THERAPISTS LIKE TO SAY, "When sex goes well it accounts for 15 percent of a marriage; but when sex is bad, it's 85 percent." The unfortunate fact is that even those of us who fall into the latter category rarely talk to our partners about sex. We have been taught that intercourse is instinctual and there is certainly no need to analyze it; good sex should come naturally. Are we naturally out of our minds? What leads us to believe that all social, intellectual and psychomotor behavior requires instruction and training, but then assume that sex does not? Our twisted morality has taught us that "novice," "innocence" and "virginal" connote an ideal female status. We are left standing on the high board about to take that first spectacular dive— with nary a swimming lesson. We risk drowning.

A license is required in order for us to drive. Although we will never get a similar certificate for sex, we can consider open dialogue and communication with our partner an unofficial endorsement of our readiness to embark on a course that will give us pleasure and expand the meaning of our union. So let's talk!

TALKING TO YOUR PARTNER

A postcoital dialogue might seem to be the best way to grade the event and discuss a score of only 4.3 with your spouse or partner. But as we all know, sex is not an Olympic sport. It doesn't warrant immediate judgment, and if we want to improve our score, we need to find a better place and time to talk. (Remember, he's not going to be very receptive to anything during his resolution period.) Most therapists recommend that a couple who wants to talk about sex find a relaxed time to sit together (somewhere other than the bedroom), hold hands or touch and establish a closeness that will not exist after a disappointing sexual experience. The conversation should not be confrontational. You are at your most vulnerable when you confess your sexual insecurities and let your partner in on your sexual needs. He responds similarly, so avoid being accusatory or didactic in your comments. Watch out for phrases such as "you always do xxx" or "you should try yyy." Better ones would be "what do I do that you like?" and "let me tell you what you do that I like." After reading the works of several excellent therapists and talking to many of my patients, here is a list of icebreakers.

10 WAYS TO TALK TO YOUR LOVER

1. "I know it can be embarrassing to talk about sex, but we're both adults."
2. "I have something to say, but I find it difficult to talk about."
3. "You may have noticed that I've been avoiding situations where we would have sex."
4. "You don't seem to be in the mood for sex lately. Is there anything you want to talk about?"
5. "Have you noticed that we've fallen into a routine when it comes to sex? Do you ever think about us being more adventurous?"
6. "Let's try making love when we're fresh, first thing in the morning—or let's plan an afternoon siesta together."
7. "It's time to send the kids to visit relatives and have a weekend to ourselves."
8. "Let's try just cuddling or giving each other a massage tonight."
9. "It's harder for me to get aroused these days. I'm not sure why, but I was hoping we could talk about it."

10. "I worry that if we try to have intercourse, I might be dry and sex will hurt."

A lot of us have been taught that in order for peace and harmony to reign in our relationship, we have to compromise. And inevitably, female compromise entails silence, compliance and surrender. We give up on getting—or never learn—what gives us pleasure. Rarely are we the initiators or the directors of the process that binds us as a couple. Although we may not consciously acknowledge it, this denial of our own needs can result in a simmering anger. Competing needs (yours and his) mean that, ultimately, sex is a power play. And if unfulfillment and anger become the predominant factors, we deny ourselves and our partner the raison d'être for sex: mutual pleasure and intimacy.

No matter how much we know or think we know about our partners, or even how much we love them, we cannot assume that mind-reading comes with the territory. Sometimes it helps to play the proverbial child's game "I'll tell if you will." Asking your partner to list the things you do that tell him you love him, and reciprocating with a similar list of your own, may be the way to make up for a lack of mental telepathy. This is not just a list of preferred sexual techniques; it's a record of all the little things he does that show you he cares, such as "I like it when you make coffee for me in the morning" and "It makes me so happy when you call me in the middle of the day to tell me you love me."

Writing lists and talking about problems helps, but you need to spend time as a couple outside the bedroom, have fun together and support each other during life's crises in order to enhance communication and intimacy. This sounds like simple common sense but it is not all that easy, particularly in two-career families with kids.

Just as taking a cold medicine will not be sufficient for most of us to overcome bacterial pneumonia, talking to our partner may not be enough to repair a damaged sexual relationship. Sometimes we need to bring in the professionals. Most of us have the sense to see a doctor if we're sick and don't get better on our own, but unfortunately, we don't apply the same principles to sex. Add to this the fact that many of us consider sexual dysfunction shameful and not a medical problem. Few of us will look in the yellow pages for a sex therapist or even for a family counselor. We should, however, feel more comfortable confiding in our doctor, who can guide us on our quest for sexual health.

TALKING TO YOUR DOCTOR

This is not as easy as it should be. We can give explicit descriptions of our periods, our bowel movements and vaginal discharge, but we find it difficult to bring up the topic of sex. In one recent study, only 3 percent of women talked to their gynecologist about sexual dysfunction during a routine visit. An additional 16 percent mentioned problems only when they were directly questioned. There seemed to be a "you don't ask, I won't tell" mentality.

While doctors focus in on your cardiovascular, digestive and reproductive systems and might even inquire "how you are doing," they are not trained to ask (nor do they always want to know), "Have you had an orgasm lately?" Many physicians find the idea of sexual history-taking uncomfortable. Just because physicians are M.D.s doesn't mean we are sexually self-assured and have reached a point in our lives where we can talk easily about sex. (This is not something that is traditionally taught in medical school.) If your doctor does not ask you if you have any sexual complaints or problems in your relationship, or whether your libido or sexual response has changed, it is up to you to introduce the subject.

One way to start this discussion is to take a copy of the sexual health checklist on page 41 with you to the office and underline those issues that you want to address. Be specific when describing physical symptoms such as vaginal dryness or pain during intercourse. This is not a time for euphemisms or vague statements such as, "Sex doesn't feel like it used to." Try to pinpoint the location, duration, onset and type of pain or discomfort, if one exists. If your libido has decreased, evaluate whether this is partner-specific or general. Don't be embarrassed to talk about masturbation—whether you are doing it, whether it turns you on or whether all attempts at stimulation have failed. Also inform your doctor of any non-sex-related changes in your health, even if they seem trivial. Make sure your doctor hears you out. Without a complete picture it will be very difficult to tease apart the possible causes of any problem.

Your physician may suggest blood tests and will certainly perform a general physical and pelvic exam. If the therapy that you are then offered includes hormone replacement, get a clear picture of the pros and cons. What can you expect it to do for your health, your symptoms and any sexual dysfunction? How fast should the treatment work? Unless you are an informed hormone consumer, you will inevitably become one of the 75 percent of women who either never fill the prescription or quickly stop taking it. One prescription does not fit all, but your doctor can't work with you unless you maintain an ongoing dialogue about your symptoms and responses.

Rarely can sexual dysfunction or hormonal imbalance be cured with one office visit. If the doctor decides to treat you with male hormones, it is clear from the preceding chapters that certain tests and follow-ups are necessary to make sure the therapy is appropriate and safe. Keep those appointments and get those tests.

Some M.D.s are not comfortable discussing the emotional and psychological impact of sexual difficulties, and there are those who may make you feel that your sexual problems are either entirely in your head or entirely in your genitals. This simplistic separation of mind and body is often dismissive and inadequate, particularly if the

"I DON'T HAVE THE RIGHT
TO ENJOY SEX"

Laurie is a 34-year-old florist. She came to see me because, with one exception, she had never experienced an orgasm and wanted to know if she had a physical or hormonal problem. This complaint was just the tip of the iceberg. Laurie is one of the most complex and troubled young women that I have ever treated. She was raised until puberty by her grandparents, who led her to believe they were actually her parents. In her early teens, her real mother showed up with a boyfriend, announced her identity and took Laurie off to live with them. At 15, Laurie was date-raped, and at 16 a boyfriend gave her herpes. Her periods started at the age of 14, but stopped for two years in her early twenties when she became anorexic. She gained some weight and her cycles returned but were not regular.

When Laurie first came to see me she was taking Desogen birth control pills and her cycles were fine. Her weight was low, but stable; she was exercising, and she had just started taking vitamins. But Laurie acknowledged that she had felt so depressed that she'd contemplated suicide. She began taking Prozac one year ago.

Laurie has problems attaching and forming relationships with men. Those she dates tend to be heavy drinkers and drug users. When Laurie is with them, she may consume up to four or five drinks. She told me she now has this bingeing down to no more than twice a month. She also mentioned that her libido is nonexistent.

After Laurie had confided this heart-wrenching history, she quietly looked at me and summarized, "I'm a mess, and

I don't know where to start. Do you?" The doctor in me started with the easy laboratory stuff—testing Laurie's blood count, liver function (to check for alcohol damage) and thyroid function. All were fine; so were her DHEAS levels. But her total testosterone was less than 10 nanograms/per deciliter (normal is 20 to 80), and her free testosterone was 0.1 picograms per nanoliter (normal is 0.8 to 3.2), so at least I could point to a possible accessory to the crime of Laurie's libido deficiency: her low bioactive male hormone. There were no fewer than three factors that contributed to this: her history of an eating disorder that may still be present as an eating "disnormalcy" (she gained back some of her weight, but her ovaries may not have completely recovered); her use of a monophasic birth control pill; and finally, the Prozac.

But that's not all, and the woman in me wants to cry because of all Laurie's other issues that, by themselves, would be ample cause for her inability to achieve orgasm or want sex—her lack of childhood trust and confidence, her sexual abuse and her chronic use of alcohol.

I started with a pharmacologic approach (which, of course, is the easiest). I suggested Wellbutrin instead of, or perhaps in addition to, her Prozac; a triphasic birth control pill instead of her current one; and testosterone propionate 2-percent ointment to be applied nightly for four weeks, then every other night thereafter. Laurie was already seeing a psychologist; I suggested she also see a sex therapist. But, mostly, I congratulated her because she had taken a lot of steps (actually, giant strides) to overcome what she termed as her "mess." She sought help, not just from me, but also from a psychotherapist.

It may take years, if not the rest of her life, for Laurie to confront, analyze and get beyond the myriad issues that have damaged her psyche and libido, but she is willing to put in the effort. Laurie wants fulfilling sex to be part of her recovery. She will return to see me in three months so we can evaluate her response. Neither she nor I expect a sudden or complete improvement; we're in this for the long term.

problem has been going on for some time. Any gynecologist worth her speculum will appreciate the emotional impact of sexual troubles and can often be the bridge that connects you with a counselor or therapist for more specialized help. Over the years, I have found that so many women approach me with emotionally charged sexual problems that in order to offer the care they need, I've added a sex therapist to my office staff. Even with this one-stop-shopping approach, I am always surprised how difficult it is for my patients to make or keep that first crucial therapy appointment. But those who do get the help they really need.

TALKING TO A SEX THERAPIST

Our society has a long-standing bias against mental health care and even today, in the much-touted age of Prozac, there are many who feel that consulting a therapist is tantamount to admitting they are "crazy." And *sex* therapy? That must *really* mean you're weird.

Drs. Jennifer Knopf and Michael Seiler, in their book *ISD: Inhibited Sexual Desire*, created a comprehensive list that will help you decide if you are likely to need professional assistance. You should seek therapy if:

- You and/or your partner have significant or persistent depression.

- You are experiencing severe marital conflicts such as abuse, arguments that don't solve problems or frequent discussion of separation or divorce.
- You routinely have conversations about sex but make no progress.
- You have a long-term sense of unhappiness or dissatisfaction with your relationship.
- You and/or your partner have an alcohol or drug problem.
- Either of you has unresolved emotional issues stemming from sexual assault, child abuse, a divorce or some type of family dysfunction.
- Your sexual relationship has never been satisfactory, or it never recovered after a period of stress in your life.
- You experience any sexual difficulties for a long period of time.
- You routinely avoid sex and/or have little or no desire for it.

WHAT HAPPENS IN SEX THERAPY?

The first visit with a sex therapist is a lot like your first visit with a new physician, except that the history-taking process may be far more exhaustive and intimate. These are the areas that the therapist will need to explore in order to help you:

- **Your health.** Do you have any health problems? What medications are you taking? What do you use for contraception? Have you had any fertility or pregnancy problems? Have you ever had a sexually transmitted disease? How did it make you feel? Do you ever feel depressed, anxious or panicky? Have you seen or do you plan to see a physician to discuss what is going on in your sex life?
- **Your family.** How did (does) it function? What kinds of attitudes were you raised with? How did your family feel about nudity, touch and expressions of affection between adults and

between parent and child? What did you perceive as your parents' level of closeness? Were gender roles divided along very traditional lines? How was anger handled? Was there abuse or domestic violence? Did any family member suffer from depression or mental health problems?

- **Your cultural and religious upbringing.** Was virginity highly valued and sex perceived as shameful? At what age were women in your family expected to become sexually active? Was sex viewed primarily as an act of procreation or one of pleasure? Did you feel you had permission to ask questions about sex?

- **What puberty was like for you.** Did your parents prepare you to go through puberty? Do you think you went through the changes of puberty at the "right" age? Did your body changes make you feel uncomfortable or unattractive?

- **Your early sexual experiences and memories.** How did you find out about sex? What was your first genital contact? Do you remember it with shame or does it evoke bad dreams? Were you sexually abused? If so, was it just touching, or did penetration occur? Was peer pressure the reason you first had intercourse? Did you do it just in order to "get it over with?" Were you taught about contraception? Did you use it? Did your sexual experiences involve drugs or alcohol? Have you ever engaged in any same-sex experimentation? What are your memories of peak erotic experiences?

- **Masturbation.** Do you masturbate? If so, when did you start? How often do you do it? Does it give you pleasure? Do you have an orgasm?

- **Eating disorders and body image issues.** Are you happy with your body? Have you ever had an eating disorder? Do you think you're fat? Have you lost or gained a lot of weight lately? Do you think your partner would like you to be thinner or heavier than you are? Do you think of yourself as sexy? Have you made changes in your body to make yourself more seductive or are there any changes you would like to make? When you imagine yourself having sex, what do you look like?

- **Fantasies.** Do you have them? Are you comfortable with them? Do you use them to enhance sexual pleasure?

The next step is to explore your current relationship. The therapist can do this with you separately or with your partner, but at some point will want to talk to each of you alone. You will be asked what you like about your relationship and what you dislike, how you met your partner, how sex was in the beginning and how it is now.

Then you'll get down to the nitty gritty: You may be given a sexual questionnaire to fill out. It will ask you what goes on during your sexual encounters. How often do you have intercourse? Who initiates? How frequently would you like to have intercourse? How often do you think about sex or feel sexual desire? How long does foreplay last? Is it long enough to get you aroused? How long does intercourse last? Is that too short a time, or too long? Does your partner experience premature ejaculation? When you have sex, do you ever feel afraid, ashamed, disgusted or guilty? Do you reach orgasm? What triggers it? Can you have an orgasm from sexual intercourse or only from clitoral stimulation? Does your partner have trouble getting or keeping an erection? Are you tight or dry? Does intercourse hurt? Would you rate your partner as a good lover? Do you think you are? How interested are you in having great sex?

These are very general questions, and others may arise depending on your answers. You and your partner (if you have one) are the only ones who can define your problem and set your goals. Don't feel you have to meet a set standard of sexual fulfillment. For some of us, the objective will simply be better understanding of one another's sexual needs. For others it may be a discovery (or rediscovery) of libido and orgasm.

Once you have articulated what you want, your therapist can begin to work with you. There are many possible approaches. I'm going to outline one that follows a distinctive, gradual pattern and is designed to guide both patient and therapist toward a solution.

THE PLISSIT PATH

PLISSIT stands for Permission, Limited Information, Specific Suggestions and Intensive Therapy. Let's look at each stage:

Permission. Before you can satisfy your sexual needs, you have to give yourself and your partner permission to fulfill them. Although these needs may seem elementary, many of us either have been brought up to deny them or have learned to repress them—for the good of our relationship, for our family, in order to conform to societal roles or because we don't feel we deserve pleasure. We have the need, even the right, to be loved and emotionally supported, to trust and be trusted, to be touched, to be sexual and to know that we are important to others. These needs are lifelong. But many of us have had our trust violated and our needs denied. We can react either by becoming soul-sufficient and self-sufficient or, conversely, by developing expectations that any sexual contact—even one that comes without intimacy—will provide the love we crave. Those of us without partners may deny our sexual needs or feel that it's pitiful to try and fulfill them by ourselves. We need permission to be sexual on our own.

Limited Information. This is the education portion of your therapy, designed to get you in touch with your own eroticism and provide you with accurate sex information. Your therapist might loan you videos, provide you with pamphlets about sex toys and paraphernalia or recommend erotic reading material. Some favorites are *The Good Vibrations Guide to Sex* and the *Good Vibrations* toy catalog, the *Lov-*

er's *Guide Encyclopedia*, *Passionate Marriage* by David Schnarch, Ph.D., and *The New Male Sexuality* by Bernie Zilbergeld. Books of erotic stories for women include *Pleasures* by Lonnie Barbach and *Forbidden Flowers* and *Women on Top* by Nancy Friday. Romance novels, soap operas and erotic films can help our imagination and allow us to become more comfortable with our fantasies.

Specific Suggestions. Most therapists agree that it is not enough for us to talk about sexual problems; we must also work on them at a physical level. Behavioral therapy techniques include homework that is done away from the therapist's office. You and your partner might be asked to schedule a trip to a store that sells seductive clothing, or one that sells sexually explicit books or sex toys. Another assignment might be to rent and watch an erotic movie together. Sometimes homework can be as simple as scheduling time together in order to facilitate closeness and communication. If relationship conflict is an issue, a couple might do a role-playing exercise in the therapist's office and then be asked to practice it at home.

Now to get to the touchy-feely part: Sensate focus exercises are often recommended to help you and your partner relax and concentrate on touching one another without sexual intent. This can start as facial or hand massages and progress to other parts of your bodies. The goal is to feel comfortable giving and receiving pleasure without having to perform or reach orgasm.

If you're comfortable with it, you might be told to become aware of your sexual responses by experimenting with masturbation. You can then share what pleases you with your partner. Several studies have shown that the overall success rate of masturbation training for women who have never been orgasmic is 90 percent or better. But if a woman who was previously orgasmic becomes unable to have an orgasm, success rates of masturbation therapy are often lower, since this problem tends to be associated with emotional issues.

Your therapist might also suggest ways to increase intimacy during sex so the act is not merely mechanical. She or he might encourage you and your partner to learn to be more sexually assertive and attempt new techniques to relieve the boredom of your sexual routine. Depending on what your goals are, you might go on to experiment with sex toys and oral sex. This is a give-and-take process and each of you should have a chance to express your interests in new techniques, but neither partner should coerce the other into behavior that he or she finds unpleasant or uncomfortable.

Intensive Therapy. If the previous steps are not sufficient, or if you and your therapist conclude that you have underlying psychiatric problems such as depression, anxiety, obsessive-compulsive disorder or bipolar disorder, more intensive therapy and possibly a consultation with a psychopharmacologist (a psychiatrist who specializes in the use of medications) is in order. Not every condition can be treated with drugs, and unresolved issues surrounding past family dysfunction, trauma, sexual abuse or rape, as well as current relationship problems, may warrant more concentrated assessment and care.

HOW TO FIND A GOOD THERAPIST

Sex therapy has become a fertile area for quacks and pseudoprofessionals. Very few states license sex therapists, so it is necessary to use the same good judgment and common sense you would use when choosing your doctor. Among the different specialists practicing sex therapy are psychologists, social workers, psychiatrists, marriage therapists and even ministers.

Ultimately, the type of shingle that a practitioner hangs out is probably less important than how comfortable you feel and how well this person does her or his job. But as a general rule, look for someone

A GOOD SEX THERAPIST WILL . . .

- Ask you if you have discussed your problem with your doctor and/or recommend that you see a doctor.
- Help you articulate and set your own goals for therapy rather than dictating what your goals should be.
- Help you analyze your behavior, looking for the subtle, unspoken messages in your sexual frequency, foreplay, arousal and orgasm (or lack thereof) rather than simply make blanket prescriptions for ways you can change your technique.
- Not attempt to impose her or his idea of what is appropriate.
- Not be afraid to make referrals when needed.

A GOOD SEX THERAPIST WON'T . . .

- Focus on the physical mechanics of sex without addressing any deeper relationship or personal psychological issues.
- Suggest you end a relationship unless you are in physical danger.
- Ask you to take off your clothes, videotape your sexual encounters or perform sexually in front of her or him.
- Insist that you do anything that makes you uncomfortable.

who is a licensed social worker, psychologist, psychiatrist or psychiatric nurse. Ideally the person will have trained in sex therapy at a teaching hospital or an institute that specializes in treating sexual dysfunction. Find out if the therapist has been certified by or belongs to one of the following groups:

- The American Association of Sex Educators, Counselors and Therapists (AASECT)
- The Society for the Scientific Study of Sex
- American Association for Marriage and Family Therapy
- Association of Social Workers
- American Psychological Association

AASECT will provide you with a list of certified professionals in your area if you send a self-addressed, stamped envelope to P.O. Box 238, Mount Vernon, Iowa, 52314-0238.

Whenever possible, ask your doctor for a referral. If you must resort to calling names you find in the phone book, ask the psychologist or social worker what her or his specialty is rather than saying, "Are you a sex therapist?" You might want to inquire into what kinds of postgraduate courses in sex therapy or the study of sexual dysfunction the therapist has taken. If you choose a therapist who does not have a medical background, that person should be working in tandem with a physician. If the therapist is a member of the clergy, she or he should be trained in pastoral counseling or mental health care.

Cost is often an issue. The fees typically range from $75 to $150 per hour. Some insurance plans will reimburse a portion of the fee for six to 12 sessions for couple and relationship issues, and perhaps more if you are diagnosed with a mental health disorder. If the prices are more than you can afford, you may be able to obtain less expensive or even free care at a community mental health center or institute where therapists are training.

There is no way of knowing how long therapy will take until it has begun. The good news is that many of us can stop very quickly once we're reassured that we have no problem—we simply have a case of unrealistic expectations. For example, couples often end up in a therapist's office because either partner thinks that the women should experience orgasm during intercourse and that climaxing during foreplay or solely as a result of clitoral stimulation is untimely and wrong. It is not; this is part of normal female sexual response. Still other couples might need more than one or two sessions, but if you are committed, do your homework and don't expect to passively get a degree in sexual mastery, six sessions might suffice. This is not a test we have to get an "A" on. Getting in the mood, sustaining that mood and fulfilling our intimate pleasure potential is its own best reward.

A PERSONAL ASIDE

THROUGHOUT THIS BOOK, I have been gender-specific in referring
to our partners or mates. It would have been confusing and grammatically difficult to use the term "he/she" every time I discussed
relationships, chemistry or sexual function. Many women have had
same-sex experiences or live in a same-sex relationship. I feel that
the terms "bisexual" and "lesbian" have more of a political than a
sexual meaning. The need for intimacy and sexual fulfillment is universal, and women in same-sex relationships can develop the same
libido problems as women who are in female-male relationships. So
except for Chapter 11, which deals with the seventh saboteur of sex
(men), all of the medical issues most of the psychological issues discussed in this book apply to all of us.

In order to write *I'm Not in the Mood*, I reviewed a large number
of books, papers and scientific studies as well as an endless mish-mosh
of "lay" publications written by guided and misguided purveyors of "I
know what will fix what sex-ails us." Despite this avid and desperate
search for information, I came to the conclusion that a lot of us are
ailing but neither we nor the medical establishment have adequately
acknowledged or addressed our needs. In this book, I have tried to
distinguish what we do know, what may work and what traditional
and additional medicine has to offer.

It wasn't easy, and the hours needed to do this (and meet my
publisher's deadline) were long. I became one of my statistics and fell
into the "I'm too exhausted to have sex" category, as I spent most of
my waking hours (outside my medical practice) reading and writing

about sex. When I titled this book in the first person, I was sort of kidding. My wonderful husband, whom I adore, only sort of got the joke.

But the stress has now passed, and I, like millions of other women, can look forward to a better future filled with intimacy and fulfillment. I've learned a lot. I hope you have too. We all deserve to declare, "I *am* in the mood."

Judith Reichman, M.D.

RESOURCES AND RECOMMENDED READINGS

Body Image and Eating Disorders

Thomas F. Cash. *What Do You See When You Look in the Mirror? Helping Yourself to a Positive Body Image.* New York: Bantam Books, 1995.

Thomas F. Cash. *The Body Image Workbook: An 8-Step Program for Learning to Like Your Looks.* Oakland, CA: New Harbinger Publications, 1997.

Evelyn Tribole and Elyse Resch. *Intuitive Eating: A Recovery Book for the Chronic Dieter: Rediscover the Pleasures of Eating and Rebuild Your Body Image.* New York: St. Martin's Press, 1996.

Cancer and Sexuality

American Cancer Society
1599 Clifton Road NE
Atlanta, GA 30329
800-227-2345
Nurses are available 24 hours to answer questions.
www.cancer.org

National Cancer Institute
Information Service
800-4-CANCER

National Coalition for Cancer Survivorship
1010 Wayne Avenue
Silver Spring, MD 20910
301-650-9127
Information on the long-term effects of cancer and cancer treatments, decisions about hormone replacement therapy after cancer, referrals to support groups.

Leslie Schover. *Sexuality and Fertility After Cancer*. New York: John Wiley & Sons, 1997.

Compounding Pharmacies

International Association of Compounding Pharmacies
P.O. Box 1365
Sugar Land, TX 77487
800-927-4227
Provides referrals to compounding pharmacies in your area.

Depression

National Alliance for the Mentally Ill
200 N. Glebe Road, Suite 1015
Arlington, VA 22203-3754
800-950-NAMI
www.nami.org
Information about depression and other mental illness and referrals to local organizations and support groups.

Erotica

Lonnie Barbach, ed. *Erotic Interludes*. New York: Plume, 1995.

Lonnie Barbach. *Pleasures*. New York: Harper Perennial, 1985.

Nancy Friday. *Forbidden Flowers*. New York: Pocket Books, 1993.

Nancy Friday. *Women on Top*. New York: Pocket Books, 1993.

Hysterectomy

Hysterectomy Educational Resources and Services Foundation
422 Bryn Mawr Avenue
Bala Cynwyd, PA 19004
610-667-7757
www.ccon.com/hers
Information and counseling on hysterectomy and its health consequences,
and on alternatives to hysterectomy and their consequences.

Herbert A. Goldfarb and Judith Greif. *The No Hysterectomy Option: Your
Body Your Choice*. New York: John Wiley & Sons, 1997.

Incontinence

National Association for Continence
P.O. Box 8310
Spartanburg, SC 29305
800-BLADDER
www.nafc.org
Educational material on incontinence and its treatment.

The Simon Foundation for Continence
P.O. Box 835
Wilmette, IL 60091
800-23-SIMON
Information packet providing information on managing incontinence.

Infertility

Resolve, Inc.
1310 Broadway
Somerville, MA 02144-1779
617-623-0744
www.resolve.org
Referrals to doctors, support for women with infertility, information about
assisted reproductive technology.

Male Sexual Dysfunction

Impotence Hotline
800-221-5517
Background information on causes and treatments of impotence; referrals to physicians who treat it.

Impotence Information Center
800-843-4315
Information on causes and cures; referrals to urologists.

Menopause

The American Menopause Foundation
350 Fifth Avenue
NY, NY 10118
212-714-2398
Brochures and newsletters on treatment of menopause symptoms.

The North American Menopause Society
P.O. Box 94527
Cleveland, OH 44101
800-774-5342
Reading list and booklets about menopause; referrals to physicians and support groups.

Painful Sex

National Vulvodynia Association
P.O. Box 4491
Silver Spring, MD 20914-4491
301-299-0775
www.nva.org
Information on the causes and treatment of vulvodynia and vulvar vestibulitis.

Vulvar Pain Foundation
P.O. Drawer 177
Graham, NC 27253
336-226-0704
www.vulvarpainfoundation.org
Information on testing and treatment for vulvar pain; access to medical journal articles and seminars.

Prescription Drugs

Complete Drug Reference. Yonkers, NY: Consumer Reports Books, 1998.

Sex and Couples Therapy

The American Association of Sex Educators, Counselors and Therapists/
Society for the Scientific Study of Sex
P.O. Box 238
Mount Vernon, IA 52314-0238
Send a self-addressed stamped envelope to receive a list of certified profes-
sionals in your area.

American Psychological Association
750 First Street NE
Washington, DC 20002-4242
202-336-5500
Referrals to state offices that can in turn refer you to practitioners in your area.

David Schnarch. *Passionate Marriage: Love, Sex and Intimacy in Emotionally
Committed Relationships.* New York: W.W. Norton & Company, 1997.

Sex Education/Information

Sexuality Information and Education Council of the U.S.
130 West 42 Street, Suite 350
New York, NY 10036-7802
212-819-9770
www.siecus.org
Extensive information on a wide range of sex topics.

Theresa L. Crenshaw. *The Alchemy of Love and Lust: How Our Sex Hormones Influence Our Relationships.* New York: Pocket Books, 1997.

Doreen Massey, ed. *Lovers' Guide Encyclopedia: The Definitive Guide to Sex and You.* New York: Thunder's Mouth Press, 1996.

Domeena Renshaw. *7 Weeks to Better Sex.* New York: Bantam Doubleday Dell, 1995.

Cathy Winks and Anne Semans. *The New Good Vibrations Guide to Sex.* San Francisco: Cleis Press, 1994.

Bernie Zilbergeld. *The New Male Sexuality.* New York: Bantam Doubleday Dell, 1993.

Adam & Eve
P.O. Box 800
Carrboro, NC 27510
919-644-1212
800-274-0333
www.aeonline.com

Eve's Garden
119 West 57 Street, #1201
New York, NY 10019-2383
212-757-8651
800-848-3837
www.evesgarden.com

Good Vibrations
1210 Valencia Street
San Francisco, CA 94110
415-974-8990
800-289-8423
www.goodvibes.com

Sex Therapy and Couples Therapy

Jack Morin. *The Erotic Mind: Unlocking the Inner Sources of Sexual Passion and Fulfillment*. New York: HarperCollins, 1995.

Gerald Schoenewolf. *The Couples' Guide to Erotic Games*. Seacaucus, NJ: Citadel Press, 1995.

Sexually Transmitted Diseases

American Social Health Association
P.O. Box 13827
Research Triangle Park, NC 27709-9940
800-227-8922 (national STD hot line; operators answer questions and send brochures)
800-230-6039 (ASHA resource center; for written educational information)

Substance Abuse

American Council on Alcoholism
2522 St. Paul Street
Baltimore, MD 21218
800-527-5344
Referrals to counseling and treatment programs.

National Drug and Alcohol Treatment Referral Service
United States Department of Health and Human Services Center for Substance Abuse Treatment
800-662-HELP
Printed material on alcohol and drug abuse and offers information on treatment and counseling options in your state.

BIBLIOGRAPHY

Chapter 1: The "Why" of Desire

Andersen, B., and J. Cyranowski. "Women's Sexuality: Behaviors, Responses and Individual Differences." *Journal of Consulting and Clinical Psychology* 63(6) (1995): 891–906.

Levin, R., and G. Wagner. "Human Vaginal Fluid: Ionic Composition and Modification by Sexual Arousal." *Journal of Physiology* 266 (1977): 62–63.

Levin, R. "The Female Orgasm—A Current Appraisal," *Journal of Psychosomatic Research* 25 (1981): 119–133.

Levin, R., and G. Wagner. "Orgasm in the Laboratory—Quantitative Studies on Duration, Intensity, Latency and Vaginal Blood Flow." *Archives of Sexual Behavior* 14 (1985): 439–449.

Levin, R. "VIP, Vagina, Clitoral and Periurethral Glans—An Update on Human Female Genital Arousal." *Experimental and Clinical Endrocinology* 98 (1991): 61–69.

Schiavi, R. "The Biology of Sexual Function." *Clinical Sexuality* 18(1) (1995): 7–21.

Chapter 2: Who's Doing It—and Not Doing It

Hite, S. *The Hite Report: A Nationwide Study of Female Sexuality*. New York: Dell Publishing, 1976.

Janus, S., and C. Janus. *The Janus Report on Sexual Behavior*. New York: John Wiley & Sons, 1994.

Michael, R. et al. *Sex in America: A Definitive Survey*. New York: Warner Books, 1995.

Rosen, R. et al. "Prevalence of Sexual Dysfunction in Women: Results of a Survey Study of 329 Women in an Outpatient Gynecological Clinic." *Journal of Sex and Marital Therapy* 19(3) (1993): 171–188.

Student, J. "No Sex Please, We're College Graduates." *American Demographics* (February 1998): 18–23.

Chapter 3: How Hormones Rule Our Moods

Adashi, E. "The Climacteric Ovary as a Functional Gonadotropin-Driven Androgen-Producing Gland." *Fertility and Sterility* 62(1) (1994): 20–27.

Bancroft, J. "Endocrinology of Sexual Function." *Clinics in Obstetrics and Gynecology* 7(2) (1980): 253–281.

Halpern, C., J. Udry, and C. Suchindran. "Testosterone Predicts Initiation of Coitus in Adolescent Females." *Psychosomatic Medicine* 59 (1997): 161–171.

Hutchinson, K. "Androgens and Sexuality." *The American Journal of Medicine* 98(suppl. 1A) (1995): 111–115.

Kirchengast, S. et al. "Decreased Sexual Interest and Its Relationship to Body Build in Postmenopausal Women." *Maturitas* 23 (1996): 63–71.

Labrie. F. et al. "Marked Decline in Serum Concentrations of Adrenal C19 Sex Steroid Precursors and Conjugated Androgen Metabolites During Aging." *Journal of Clinical Endocrinology and Metabolism* 82(5) (1997): 2396–2402.

Leitenberg, H., M. Detzer, and D. Strebnik. "Gender Differences in Masturbation and the Relation of Masturbation Experience in Preadolescence and/ or Early Adolescence to Sexual Behavior and Sexual Adjustment in Adulthood." *Archives of Sexual Behavior* 22(2) (1993): 87–98.

Luthold, W. et al. "Serum Testosterone Fractions in Women: Normal and Abnormal Clinical States." *Metabolism* 42(5) (1993): 638–643.

Meston, C. "Aging and Sexuality." *The Western Journal of Medicine* 167(4) (1997): 285.

Rako, S. *The Hormone of Desire: The Truth About Sexuality, Menopause & Desire*. New York: Harmony Books, 1996.

Reamy, K. et al. "Sexuality and Pregnancy: A Prospective Study." *The Journal of Reproductive Medicine* 27(6) (1982): 322–327.

Reichman, J., *I'm Too Young to Get Old: Health Care for Women After Forty*, New York: Times Books, 1996.

Santoro, N., "Hormonal Changes in the Perimenopause." *Clinical Consultations in Obstetrics and Gynecology* 8(1) (1996): 2–8.

Sarrel, P. "Sexuality and Menopause." *Obstetrics and Gynecology* 75(suppl. 4) (1990): 26– 30.

Schreiner-Engel, P. et al. "Low Sexual Desire in Women: The Role of Reproductive Hormones." *Hormones and Behavior* 23 (1989): 221–234.

Sherwin, B. "Menopause: Myths and Realities." In *Psychological Aspects of Women's Health Care: The Interface Between Psychiatry and Obstetrics and Gynecology*, edited by Donna Stewart and Nada Stotland. Washington, DC: American Psychiatric Press, 1993.

Sherwin, B., and T. Owett. "The Female Androgen Deficiency Syndrome." *Journal of Sex and Marital Therapy* 19(1) (1993): 3–24.

Zumoff, B. et al. "Twenty-Four-Hour Mean Plasma Testosterone Concentration Declines with Age in Normal Premenopausal Women." *Journal of Clinical Endocrinology* 80(4) (1995): 1429–1430.

Chapter 4: "I'm Not in the Mood . . ."

Alexander, B. "Disorders of Sexual Desire: Diagnosis and Treatment of Decreased Libido." *American Family Physician* 47(4) (1993): 832– 839.

American Psychiatric Association. *Diagnostic and Statistical Manual of Mental Disorders*, 4th ed. Washington, DC: American Psychiatric Association, 1994.

Barbach, L. "Loss of Sexual Desire." *Menopause Management* January/February 1998: 10–14.

Beck, J. "Hypoactive Sexual Desire Disorder: An Overview." *Journal of Consulting and Clinical Psychology*, 63(6) (1995): 919–923.

Donahey, K., and R. Carroll. "Gender Differences in Factors Associated with Hypoactive Sexual Desire." *Journal of Sex & Marital Therapy* 19(1) (1993): 25–39.

Ernst, C., M. Földényl, and J. Angst. "The Zurich Study: XXI. Sexual Dysfunctions and Disturbances In Young Adults." *European Archives of Psychiatry and Clinical Neuroscience* 243 (1993): 179–188.

Rosen, R., and S. Leiblum. "Hypoactive Sexual Desire." *Clinical Sexuality* 18(1) (1995): 107–121.

Santoro, N. "Hormonal Changes in the Perimenopause." *Clinical Consultations in Obstetrics and Gynecology* 8(1) (1996): 2–8.

Chapter 5: Psychological Issues

Chatel, A. et al. "Psychological Distress and Sexuality in a Group of Women Attending a Menopause Clinic: Effect of Hormonal Replacement Therapy."

Menopause: The Journal of the North American Menopause Society 3(3) (1996): 165–171.

Fontana, A., and R. Rosenheck. "Duty-Related and Sexual Stess in the Etiology of PTSD Among Women Veterans Who Seek Treatment." *Psychiatric Services* 49(5) (1998): 658–662.

Herbert, J. "Sexuality, Stress and the Chemical Architecture of the Brain." *Annual Review of Sexual Research* 7 (1996): 1–43.

Herer, E., and S. Holzapfel. The Medical Causes of Infertility and Their Effects on Sexuality. *The Canadian Journal of Human Sexuality* 2(3) (1993): 113–120.

McEwen, B. "Protective and Damaging Effects of Stress Mediators." *The New England Journal of Medicine* 338(3) (1998): 171–179.

Morokoff, P. and R. Gillillan. "Stress, Sexual Functioning, and Marital Satisfaction." *The Journal of Sex Research* 30(1) (1993): 43–53.

Sarwer, D., and J. Durlak. "Childhood Sexual Abuse as a Predictor of Adult Female Sexual Dysfunction: A Study of Couples Seeking Sex Therapy." *Child Abuse & Neglect* 20(10) (1996): 963–972.

Sato, Y. et al. "Effects of Long-term Psychological Stress on Sexual Behavior and Brain Catecholamine Levels." *Journal of Andrology* 17(2) (1996): 83–90.

Stein, M. et al. "Enhanced Dexamethasone Suppression of Plasma Cortisol in Adult Women Traumatized by Childhood Sexual Abuse." *Biological Psychiatry* 42 (1997): 680–686.

Chapter 6: Couple Trouble

McCarthy, B. "Sexual Dysfunctions and Dissatisfactions Among Middle-Years Couples." *Journal of Sex Education and Therapy* 9–12 (1984).

Sprecher, S. et al. "Domains of Expressive Interaction in Intimate Relationships: Associations with Satisfaction and Commitment," *Family Relations* 44(2) (1995): 203–210.

Chapter 7: Medications

Anonymous. "Drugs That Cause Sexual Dysfunction: An Update." *The Medical Letter on Drugs and Therapeutics* 34(876) (1992).

Anonymous. *Physicians' Desk Reference 1998*, 52nd ed. Montvale, NJ: Medical Economics Data, 1997.

Balon, R., "Intermittent Amantadine for Fluoxetine-Induced Anorgasmia." *Journal of Sex and Marital Therapy* 22(4) (1996): 290–292.

Bancroft, J. et al. "Androgens and Sexual Behavior in Women Using Oral Contraceptives." *Clinical Endrocrinology* 12 (1980): 327–340.

Beckman, L., and K. Ackerman. "Women, Alcohol and Sexuality." *Recent Developments in Alcoholism* 12 (1995): 267–285.

Ferrini, R., and E. Barrett-Connor. "Caffeine Intake and Endogenous Sex Steroid Levels in Postmenopausal Women." *American Journal of Epidemiology* 144(7) (1996): 642–644.

Gitlin, M. "Psychotropic Medications and Their Effects on Sexual Function: Diagnosis, Biology and Treatment Approaches." *Journal of Clinical Psychiatry* 55(9) (1994): 406–413.

Graham, C., and B. Sherwin. "The Relationship Between Mood and Sexuality in Women Using an Oral Contraceptive as a Treatment for Premenstrual Symptoms." *Psychoneuroimmunology* 18(4) (1993): 273–281.

Hollander, E., and A. McCarley. "Yohimbine Treatment of Sexual Side Effects Induced by Serotonin Reuptake Blockers." *Journal of Clinical Psychiatry* 53(6) (1992): 207–209.

Jacobsen, F. "Fluoxetine-Induced Sexual Dysfunction and an Open Trial of Yohimbine." *Journal of Clinical Psychiatry* 53(94) (1992): 119–122.

Khaw, K. et al. "Cigarette Smoking and Levels of Adrenal Androgens in Postmenopausal Women." *The New England Journal of Medicine* 318(26) (1998): 1705–1709.

Meston, C., B. Gorzalka, and J. Wright. "Inhibition of Subjective and Physiological Sexual Arousal in Women by Clonidine." *Psychosomatic Medicine* 59(4) (1997): 399–407.

Rothschild, A. "Selective Serotonin Reuptake Inhibitor-Induced Sexual Dysfunction: Efficacy of a Drug Holiday." *American Journal of Psychiatry* 152(10) (1995): 1514–1516.

Walker, P. et al. "Improvement in Fluoxetine-Associated Sexual Dysfunction in Patients Switched to Buproprion." *Journal of Clinical Psychiatry* 54(12) (1993): 459–465.

Wilsnack, S. et al. "Predicting Onset and Chronicity of Women's Problem Drinking: A Five-Year Longitudinal Analysis." *American Journal of Public Health* 81(3) (1991): 305–318.

Chapter 8: Diseases

Curry, S. et al. "The Impact of Systemic Lupus Erythematosus on Women's Sexual Functioning." *The Journal of Rheumatology* 21(12) (1994): 2254–2260.

Dunning, P., R. Grad, and H. Dip. "Sexuality and Women with Diabetes." *Patient Education and Counseling* 21 (1993): 5–14.

Nosek, M. et al. "Sexual Functioning Among Women with Physical Disabilities." *Archives of Physical Medicine and Rehabilitation* 77 (1996): 107–115.

Perone, N. "Female Urinary Incontinence Associated with Orgasm." *Medical Aspects of Human Sexuality* (February 1998): 23–24.

Tardif, G. "Sexual Activity After a Myocardial Infarction." *Archives of Physical Medicine and Rehabilitation* 70(10) (1989): 763–766.

Chapter 9: Surgery, Chemotherapy and Radiation

Bellerose, S., and Y. Binik. "Body Image and Sexuality in Oopherectomized Women." *Archives of Sexual Behavior* 22(5) (1993): 435–459.

Corney, R. et al. "Psychosexual Dysfunction in Women with Gynaecological Cancer Following Radical Pelvic Surgery." *British Journal of Obstetrics and Gynaecology* 100 (1993): 73–78.

Hasson, H. "Cervical Removal at Hysterectomy for Benign Disease: Risks and Benefits." *Journal of Reproductive Medicine* 38(10) (1993): 781–790.

Kaplan, H. "A Neglected Issue: The Sexual Side Effects of Current Treatments for Breast Cancer." *Journal of Sex & Marital Therapy* 18(1) (1992): 3–19.

Nathorst-Boos, J., T. Fuchs, and B. von Schoultz. "Consumer's Attitude to Hysterectomy." *Acta Obstetricia et Gynecologica Scandinavica* 71 (1992): 230–234.

Ryan, M. "Hysterectomy: Social and Psychosexual Aspects." *Baillière's Clinical Obstetrics and Gynaecology* 11(1) (1997): 23–26.

Shover, L. *Sexuality and Fertility After Cancer*, New York: John Wiley & Sons, 1997.

Thranov, I., and M. Klee. "Sexuality Among Gynecologic Cancer Patients— A Cross-Sectional Study." *Gynecologic Oncology* 52 (1994): 14–19.

Zussman, L. et al. "Sexual Response After Hysterectomy-Oopherectomy: Recent Studies and Reconsideration of Psychogenesis." *American Journal of Obstetrics and Gynecology* 140(7) (1981): 725–730.

Chapter 10: Pain

Friedrich, E. and P. Kalra. "Serum Levels of Sex Hormones in Vulvar Lichen Sclerosus, and the Effect of Topical Testosterone." *The New England Journal of Medicine* 310(8) (1984): 488–491.

Meana, M. et al. "Dyspareunia: Sexual Dysfunction or Pain Syndrome?" *The Journal of Nervous and Mental Disease* 185(9) (1997): 561–569.

Paavonen, J. "Vulvodynia: A Complex Syndrom of Vulvar Pain." *Acta Obstetricia et Gynecologica Scandinavica* 74 (1995): 243–247.

Rosen, R., and S. Leiblum. "Treatment of Sexual Disorders in the 1990s: An Integrated Approach." *Journal of Consulting and Clinical Psychology* 63(6) (1995): 877–890.

Steege, J., and F. Ling. "Dyspareunia: A Special Type of Chronic Pelvic Pain." *Obstetrics and Gynecology Clinics of North America* 20(4) (1993): 779–793.

Chapter 11: The Seventh Saboteur: Men

Anonymous. "Full Prescribing Information, Viagra (sildenafil citrate) Tablets." New York: Pfizer Inc., 1998.

Goldstein, I. et al. for the Sildenafil Study Group. "Oral Sildenafil in the Treatment of Erectile Dysfunction." *The New England Journal of Medicine* 338(20) (1998): 1397–1405.

Mann, A. "Cross-Gender Sex Pill." *Time,* April 6, 1998, p. 62.

NIH Consensus Development Panel on Impotence. "Impotence." *Journal of the American Medical Association* 270(1) (1993): 83–90.

Schiavi, R., and J. Rehman. "Sexuality and Aging." *Urological Clinics of North America* 22(4) (1995): 711–726.

Utiger, R: "A Pill for Impotence?" *The New England Journal of Medicine* 338(20) (1998): 1458–1459.

Chapter 12: Testosterone and Beyond: Our Newest Hormone Replacement Options

Barnhart, K. "Is There Evidence to Replace DHEA Sulfate in Aging Men and Women?" *Menopausal Medicine* 5(3) (1997): 6–12.

Barrett-Connor, E., K. Khaw, and S. Yen. "A Prospective Study of Dehydroepiandrosterone Sulfate, Mortality and Cardiovascular Disease." *The New England Journal of Medicine* 315(24) (1986): 1519–1524.

Barrett-Connor, E. et al. "Interim Safety Analysis of a Two-Year Study Comparing Oral Estrogen-Androgen and Conjugated Estrogens in Surgically Menopausal Women." *Journal of Women's Health* 5 (1996): 593–602.

Bhasin, S., and W. Bremner. "Emerging Issues in Androgen Replacement Therapy." *Journal of Clinical Endocrinology and Metabolism* 82(1) (1997): 3–8.

Booij, A. et al. "Androgens as Adjuvant Treatment in Postmenopausal Female Patients with Rheumatoid Arthritis." *Annals of the Rheumatic Diseases* 55 (1996): 811–815.

Buster, J. et al. "Postmenopausal Steroid Repalcement with Micronized Dehydroepiandrosterone: Preliminary Oral Bioavailability and Dose Proportionality Studies." *American Journal of Obstetrics and Gynecology* 166 (1992): 1163–1170.

Casson, P. et al. "Oral Dehydroepiandrosterone in Physiological Disease Modulates Immune Function in Postmenopausal Women." *American Journal of Obstetrics and Gyneocology* 169(6) (1993): 1536–1539.

Casson, P. et al. "Replacement of Dehydroepiandrosterone Enhances T-lymphocyte Insulin Binding in Postmenopausal Women. *Fertility and Sterility* 63(5) (1995): 1027–1031.

Demers, L. "Biochemistry and Laboratory Measurement of Androgens in Women." In *Androgenic Disorders*, edited by G. P. Redmond. New York: Raven Press, Ltd., 1995, pp. 21–34.

Derman, R. "Effects of Sex Steroids on Women's Health: Implications for Practitioners." *The American Journal of Medicine* 98(suppl 1A) (1995): 137–143.

Geisthövel, F. et al. "Obesity and Hypertestosteronaemia Are Independently and Synergistically Associated with Elevated Insulin Concentrations and Dyslipidaemia in Premenopausal Women." *Human Reproduction* 9(4) (1994): 610–616.

Gelfand, M. "Estrogen-Androgen Hormone Replacement Therapy." *European Menopause Journal* 2(3) (1995): 22–26.

Gelfand, M., and B. Wiita. "Androgen and Estrogen-Androgen Hormone Replacement Therapy: A Review of the Safety Literature, 1941–1996." *Clinical Therapeutics* 19(4) (1997): 383–404.

Haffner, S., and R. Valdez. "Endogenous Sex Hormones: Impact on Lipids, Lipoproteins and Insulin." *The American Journal of Medicine* 98(suppl 1A) (1995): 40–47.

Haffner, S. et al. "Relation of Sex Hormones and Dehydroepiandrosterone Sulfate to Cardiovascular Risk Factors in Postmenopausal Women. *American Journal of Epidemiology* 142(9) (1995): 925–934.

Hickok, L., C. Toomey, and L. Speroff. "A Comparison of Esterified Estrogens with and Without Methyltestosterone: Effects on Endometrial Histology and Serum Lipoproteins in Postmenopausal Women." *Obstetrics and Gynecology* 82(6) (1993): 919–924.

Holte, J. "Disturbances in Insulin Secretion and Sensitivity in Women with the Polycystic Ovary Syndrome." *Baillieres Clinical Endocrinology and Metabolism* 10(2) (1996): 221–247.

Honoré, E. et al. "Methyltestosterone Does Not Diminish the Beneficial Effects of Estrogen Replacement Therapy on Coronary Artery Reactivity in Cynomolgus Monkeys." *Menopause: The Journal of The North American Menopause Society* 3(1) (1996): 20–26.

Insler, V., and B. Lunenfeld. "Pathophysiology of Polycystic Ovary Disease: New Insights." *Human Reproduction* 6(8) (1991): 1025–1029.

Kaplan, H., and T. Owett. "The Female Androgen Deficiency Syndrome." *Journal of Sex & Marital Therapy* 19(1) (1993): 3–24.

Karydas, I. et al. "Adjuvant Androgen Treatment of Operable Breast Cancer—A 20-Year Analysis." *European Journal of Surgical Oncology* 13 (1987): 113–117.

Kaunitz, A. "The Role of Androgens in Menopausal Hormonal Replacement." *Menopause and Hormone Replacement Therapy* 26(2) (1997): 391–397.

Labrie, F. et al. "Effect of 12-Month Dehydroepiandrosterone Replacement Therapy on Bone, Vagina and Endometrium in Postmenopausal Women." *Journal of Clinical Endrocinology and Metabolism* 82(10) (1997): 3498–3505.

Labrie, F. et al. "Physiological Changes in Dehydroepiandrosterone Are Not Reflected by Serum Levels of Active Androgens and Estrogens but of Their Metabolites: Intracrinology." *Journal of Clinical Endocrinology and Metabolism* 82(8) (1997): 2403–2409.

LaRosa, J. "Androgens and Women's Health: Genetic and Epidemiologic Aspects of Lipid Metabolism." *The American Journal of Medicine* 98(suppl 1A) (1995): 22–26.

Morales, A. et al. "Effects of Replacement Dose of Dehydroepiandrosterone in Men and Women of Advancing Age." *Journal of Clinical Endrocinology and Metabolism* 78(6) (1994): 1360– 1367.

North American Menopause Society Roundtable Highlights. "Physiologic Androgen Replacement in Menopausal Women." *Menopause Management* March/April 1998, 26–28.

Phillips, G., B. Pindernell, and T. Jing. "Relationship Between Serum Sex Hormones and Coronary Artery Disease in Postmenopausal Women." *Arteriosclerosis, Thrombosis and Vascular Biology* 17(4) (1997): 695–701.

Rittmaster, R. "Clinical Relevance of Testosterone and Dihydrotestosterone Metabolism in Women." *The American Journal of Medicine* 98(suppl 1A) (1995): 17–21.

Rosenberg, M., R. King, and C. Timmons. "Estrogen-Androgen for Hormone Replacement: A Review." *The Journal of Reproductive Medicine* 42(7) (1997): 394–402.

Sands, R., and J. Studd. "Exogenous Androgens in Postmenopausal Women." *The American Journal of Medicine.* 98(suppl 1A) (1995): 76–79.

Sherwin, B., and M. Gelfand. "Differential Symptom Response to Parenteral Estrogen and/or Androgen Administration in the Surgical Menopause." *American Journal of Obstetrics and Gynecology* 151(2) (1985): 153–160.

Sherwin B., M. Gelfand., and W. Brender. "Androgen Enhances Sexual Motivation in Females: A Prospective, Crossover Study of Sex Steroid Administration in the Surgical Menopause." *Psychosomatic Medicine* 47(4) (1985): 339–351.

Sherwin, B., and M. Gelfand. "Sex Steroids and Affect in the Surgical Menopause: A Double-Blind, Cross-Over Study." *Psychoneuroimmunology* 10(3) (1985): 325–335.

Sherwin, B. "Affective Changes with Estrogen and Androgen Replacement Therapy in Surgically Menopausal Women." *Journal of Affective Disorders* 14 (1988): 177–187.

Shoupe, D., and R. Lobo. "The Influence of Androgens on Insulin Resistance." *Fertility and Sterility* 41(3) (1984): 385–388.

University of California San Diego School of Medicine. "The Emerging Role of Estrogen/Androgen Therapy in the Care of the Postmenopausal Patient," a CME monograph highlighting presentation from an educational symposium held during the XV FIGO World Congress of Gynecology and Obstetrics, August 1997.

Urman, B., S. Pride, and B. Yuen. "Elevated Serum Testosterone, Hirsutism and Virilism Associated with Combined Androgen-Estrogen Hormone Replacement Therapy. *Obstetrics and Gynecology* 77(4) (1991): 595–598.

Watts, N. et al. "Comparison of Oral Estrogens and Estrogens Plus Androgen on Bone Mineral Density, Menopausal Symptoms, and Lipid-Lipoprotein Profiles in Surgical Menopause." *Obstetrics and Gynecology* 85(4) (1995): 529–537.

Wild, R. "Obesity, Lipids, Cardiovascular Risk and Androgen Excess." *The American Journal of Medicine* 98(suppl 1A) (1995): 27–32.

Chapter 13: More Than Hormones: Alternatives and Adjuncts

Azar, B. "Communicating Through Pheremones." *American Psychological Association Monitor* 29(1) (1998): 1–12.

Choi, H., D. Seong, and K. Rha. "Clinical Efficacy of Korean Red Ginseng for Erectile Dysfunction." *International Journal of Impotence Research* 7(3) (1995): 181–186.

Hirsch, A. *Scentsational Sex: The Secret to Using Aroma for Arousal.* Rockport, MA: Element Books, 1998.

Kim, C. et al. "Influence of Ginseng on Mating Behavior of Male Rats." *American Journal of Chinese Medicine* 4(2) (1976):163–168.

Lasalandra, M., "Ride May Be Over for Some Cyclists." *The Boston Herald,* September 18, 1997, p. 29.

Lindgren, R. et al. "Effects of Ginseng on Quality of Life in Postmenopausal Women" (Free communication, annual meeting). *North American Menopause Society,* 1997.

Meston, C., and B. Gorzalka. "Differential Effects of Sympathetic Activation on Sexual Arousal in Sexually Dysfunctional and Functional Women." *Journal of Abnormal Psychology* 105(4) (1996): 582–591.

Meston, C., and B. Gorzalka. "The Effects of Immediate, Delayed, and Residual Sympathetic Activation on Sexual Arousal in Women." *Behavioral Research Therapeutics* 34(2) (1996): 143–148.

Nordenberg, T. "From Anchovies to Oysters: Do Aphrodisiacs Really Work?" *FDA Consumer,* January–February 1996.

Rosen, R., and A. Ashton. "Prosexual Drugs: Empirical Status of the 'New Aphrodisiacs.'" *Archives of Sexual Behavior,* 22(6) 1993: 521–543.

Segraves, R. "Pharmacological Enhancement of Human Sexual Behavior." *Journal of Sex Education and Therapy* 17(4) (1991): 283–289.

Chapter 14: Can We Talk?

Annon, J. "The Behavioral Treatment of Sexual Problems." In *Brief Therapy,* New York: Harper & Row, 1976.

Barbach, L. *For Yourself.* New York: Signet Books, 1976.

Crenshaw, T. *The Alchemy of Love and Lust: How Our Sex Hormones Influence Our Relationships.* New York: Pocket Books, 1997.

Hales, D. "The Joy of Midlife Sex." *American Health for Women* (January/ February 1997): 78–81.

Heiman, J., and J. Lopiccolo. *Becoming Orgasmic: A Sexual Growth Program for Women*. New York: Simon & Schuster/Fireside, 1986.

Hurlbert, D. "A Comparative Study Using Orgasm Consistency Training in the Treatment of Women Reporting Hypoactive Sexual Desire." *Journal of Sex & Marital Therapy* 19(1) (1993): 41–55.

Kaplan, H. *The New Sex Therapy*. New York: Random House, 1974.

Knopf, J., and M. Seiler. *ISD: Inhibited Sexual Desire*. New York: William Morrow & Company, Inc., 1990.

Massey, D., ed. *Lovers' Guide Encyclopedia: The Definitive Guide to Sex and You,* New York: Thunder's Mouth Press, 1996.

Morin, J. *The Erotic Mind: Unlocking the Inner Sources of Sexual Passion and Fulfillment,* New York: HarperCollins, 1995.

O'Donohue, W., C. Dopke, and D. Swingen. "Psychotherapy for Female Sexual Dysfunction: A Review." *Clinical Psychology Review* 17(5) (1997): 537–566.

Offit, A. *The Sexual Self*. Philadelphia: J. B. Lippincott Co., 1977.

Rosen, R., and S. Lieblum. *Principles and Practice of Sex Therapy: Update for the 1990's,* 2nd ed. New York: The Guilford Press, 1989.

Rosen, R., and S. Lieblum. *Case Studies in Sex Therapy*. New York: The Guilford Press, 1995.

Schnarch, D. *Constructing the Sexual Crucible: An Integration of Sexual and Mental Therapy*. New York: W.W. Norton & Company, 1991.

Schnarch, D. *Passionate Marriage: Love, Sex and Intimacy in Emotionally Committed Relationships*. New York: W.W. Norton & Company, 1997.

Watson, J., and T. Davies. "Psychosexual Problems: ABCs of Mental Health." *British Medical Journal* 315(7102) (1997): 239.

Zilbergeld, Bernie.*The New Male Sexuality*. New York: Bantam Books, 1992.

INDEX

AASECT (American Association of Sex Educators, Counselors and Therapists), 155, 156
acne, 63, 70, 109, 117, 120, 124
adrenal glands, 24–25, 31, 53, 105, 106, 125
adrenarche, 24
adrenopause, 126
age factors:
  in breast surgery, 86–87
  in DHEA levels, 126
  in diminished libido, 4
  in frequency of intercourse, 18
  in frequency of masturbation, 20
  in frequency of orgasm, 19
  in hormonal levels, 30–31
  in male erectile dysfunction, 94, 97–98
  in perimenopause, 30–31
  in SHBG levels, 31
  in testosterone levels, 106
  in weight gain, 54
albumin, 27
alcohol, see drinking
Alesse, 63
allergy remedies, 71
alprazolam, 69
alprostadil (Caverjet; Edex; Muse Pellet), 98
Alzheimer's disease, 65, 125
amantadine (Symmetrel), 67–68
American Association for Marriage and Family Therapy, 156
American Association of Sex Educators, Counselors and Therapists (AASECT), 155, 156
American Health for Women, 37, 54
American Psychiatric Association, 38, 39
American Psychological Association, 156
amino acids, 139
amitriptyline, 67
Anaprox (Naproxen), 71
anatomy, 14–16
androgens, see male hormones

androstendione, 25–27
anemia, test for, 118
anger, reactions to, 57–58
anorexia, 53
antacids, 71
anti-anxiety medications, 96, 113
antibiotics, 71, 89
anticholesterol medications, 71
anticonvulsants, 69
antidepressants, 48–49, 54, 62, 66–69, 96, 100, 113, 131, 134, 135
anti-epileptic medications, 69, 71, 76–77
antifungal medications, 71
antihistamines, 68, 71
antihormones, 65–66
anti-inflammatories, 71
antioxidants, 139
antipsychotics, 68, 96, 100
antispasmodic drugs, 78
anxiety, 47, 49–51, 95
aphrodisiacs, 129–133
Aphrodite, 129
Aphrodyne (yohimbine hydrochloride), 131
apomorphine (Spontane), 133
areola, 11
arteriosclerosis, 95
arthritis, 75, 108
Association of Social Workers, 154
Astroglide, 137
atherosclerosis, 110
autoimmune diseases, 75–76
Axid (nizatidine), 71

barbiturates, 72
bee pollen, 131
behavioral therapy, 153
benzodiazepines, 69
beta-blocking drugs, 70
bicycling, 138
birth control pills, 52–54, 62–64, 93, 113, 146, 147

185

black cohosh (Remifemin), 132
bladder, 89, 92
bleeding, control of, 65
bloating, 64, 70
blood pressure, *see* hypertension
blood sugar levels, 73
body hair, excess, 26, 70, 105, 109–110, 120, 124
body image, 53–55
bone marrow transplant, 82
bones, 107–108, 139
boys, *see* males
brain, 5, 9, 12, 16, 25, 49
breast cancer, 5, 82, 86–87, 112, 117
    polycystic ovarian syndrome and, 105
    SERMs and, 64
breast-feeding, 4, 29–30
breasts:
    development of, 24
    reconstruction of, 86
    surgery and, 86–87
    tenderness of, 108
bromocriptine (Parlodel), 134
bulimia, 53
buproprion (Wellbutrin; Zyban), 67, 135, 140, 147
BuSpar, 69

caffeine, 72
calcium, 89, 139
cancer, 4–5, 74, 127
    colon, 65
    liver, 112
    ovarian, 4
    prostate, 125
    treatment of, 80–81
    uterine, 105, 112
    see also breast cancer
cardiovascular disease, 5, 65, 74
    DHEA and, 125, 126
    eating disorders and, 54
    hormone therapy and, 110–111
    male erectile dysfunction and, 95–96, 97, 100
    polycystic ovarian syndrome and, 105
    testosterone therapy and, 116, 117
Caverjet (alprostadil), 98
central nervous system, 69–70
cervix, 11, 84–86
chemical attraction, relationships and, 58–60
chemical menopause, 65
chemotherapy, 81–82, 86
childhood sexual abuse, 51
Chinese tea tree, 132
chlordiazepoxide, 69
chlorpromazine, 68

chlorprothixine, 68
chocolate, 131
cholesterol, 97, 110–111, 116, 126
    medications for, 71
    profile of, 118, 124
chronic stress, 49
cimetidine (Tagamet), 71
climax, *see* orgasm
clitoris, 11, 13–14
    Desyrel and, 67
    testosterone and, 27, 36, 113, 121
clitoromegaly, 109, 110
clobetasol, 92
clonazepam (Klonopin), 69
clonidine, 70
cocaine, 72
coffee, 72
cold remedies, 71
collagen, 75
colognes, 136
colon cancer, 65
communication and dialogue:
    with doctor, 144–148
    with partner, 58, 141–144
    with sex therapist, 148–154
compounding pharmacies, 120, 122–123, 128
compression fractures, spinal, 139
conservatives, sexual activity of, 21
contraceptives, oral, *see* birth control pills
corpus luteum, 25
corticosteroid drugs, 75
cortisol, 48
couples, frequency of intercourse of, 18
cranberry tablets, 92
cryosurgery, 89
Cushing's syndrome, 106
cyclic guanosine monophosphate (cyclic GMP), 99, 100
Cycrin (medroxyprogesterone acetate), 34, 64
cyproheptadine (Perioactin), 68
cystitis, 89
cystocele, 78
cysts, 81, 92

damiana, 132
Danazol, 66
dehydroepiandrosterone (DHEA), 25–27, 124–128
dehydroepiandrosterone sulfate (DHEAS), 25, 118, 125
dehydrotestosterone (DHT), 26, 139–140
Demulen, 52, 63, 64
Depakote (valproic acid), 69, 70, 77
Depo-Provera, 63
deprenyl (Eldepryl), 134
depression, 146, 148

chemotherapy and, 81
hysterectomy and, 85
libido and, 28, 66
lupus and, 75
male erectile dysfunction and, 95
as medical side effect, 64
medications for, 48–49, 54, 62, 66–69, 96,
    100, 113, 131, 134, 135
postpartum, 29
serotonin and, 66
sexual abuse and, 51
testosterone and, 36, 107
designer estrogens, 64
desipramine, 67
Desogen, 63, 146
Desyrel (trazadone), 67, 135
DHEA (dehydroepiandrosterone), 25–27,
    124–128
DHEAS (DHEA sulfate), 25, 118, 125
DHT (dehydrotestosterone), 26, 139–140
diabetes, 54–55, 73, 95, 100, 105, 116
*Diagnostic and Statistical Manual of Mental
    Disorders*, 38
diet, 50, 53, 70, 97, 139
digoxin, 70
Dilantin (phenytoin), 71
disulfuram, 71
Ditropan, 78
diuretics, 70
divorce, 40, 56, 58
dominance, 47
dong quai, 132–133
dopamine, 48, 66, 68, 70, 133, 134
doxepin, 67
drinking, 20, 71–72, 97, 146, 149
drowsiness, 65, 68, 71
drug holiday, 67
drugs, recreational, *see* substance abuse
drugs, therapeutic, *see* medications
dyspareunia, *see* painful intercourse

eating disorders, 53–54, 146, 147
echinacea, 132
Edex (alprostadil), 98
education, sexual activity and, 21
egg, development of, 25, 30
Eldepryl (deprenyl), 134
Elders, Joycelyn, 20
endometriosis, 65, 66, 81, 88, 92
endometrium, 25
endorphins, 138
    receptors of, 9
energy levels, 49, 107
epilepsy, 69, 71, 76–77
episiotomy, 29
erectile dysfunction:

in men, 29, 73, 94–100, 131–133, 134
in women, 61, 68–71, 77
Erex (yohimbine hydrochloride), 132
erotic reading material, 152–153
estradiol, 115, 123
Estratab, 120
Estratest, 109, 119–120
Estratest H.S., 120, 122
Estring, 82, 84, 115
estrogen, 3, 24–25, 27, 30
    antihormones and loss of, 65
    in birth control pills, 62
    bone density and, 108
    breast cancer and, 5
    chemotherapy and, 81
    creams, 84, 115
    depression and, 48–49
    designer, 64
    DHEA and, 125
    eating disorders and, 54
    fat distribution and, 24
    menopause and, 31–32
    methyltestosterone and, 119–120
    obesity and, 54
    painful intercourse and, 88, 93
    patches, 82, 84, 123
    perimenopausal levels of, 31
    plants, 132–133
    postpartum decline, 30
    prolactin and, 29
    receptors, 9
    sexual arousal and, 11
    SHBG production and, 27
    testosterone and, 117, 119
    weight loss and levels of, 53
estrogen therapy, 23, 32, 34, 35, 64–65, 123
    after breast cancer, 82
    diminished libido and, 4
    with GnRH analogs, 66
    heart disease and, 110
    menopausal symptoms and, 108
    in multiple sclerosis, 76
    after oopherectomy, 83–84
    for stress incontinence, 78
    for vaginal dryness, 137
Evista (raloxifene), 64, 115
exercise, 50, 70, 74, 97, 138–139
exhibitionism, 47
extramarital affairs, 21, 50, 58

famotidine (Pepcid), 71
fat cells, hormone production in, 26, 33, 54
fat distribution, estrogen and, 24
fatigue, 49, 53–54, 81, 107
females, 2
    DHEA in, 125

females (*cont.*)
  eating disorders in, 53
  heart attacks in, 111
  incidence of depression in, 48
  male hormones in, 10, 24, 27–28
  medical side effects in, 61
  pubescent girls, 10, 27–28
  reaction to anger by, 57
  sexual disorders in, 40; *see also specific*
    disorders
  stress in, 49
  testosterone and, 27–28
Fem-Patch, 82
Ferrare, Christina, 2–3
fibroids, 65, 81, 92
fight-or-flight response, 49
first bypass, 119–120, 128
folic acid, 139
follicles, ovarian, 25–26, 30–31
follicle stimulating hormone (FSH), 25, 26,
    48, 65, 118
formulating pharmacies, *see* compounding
    pharmacies
Freud, Sigmund, 47
FSH (follicle stimulating hormone), 25, 26,
    48, 65, 118

gemfibrozil (Lopid), 71
genitalia, 14–16
  diabetes and, 73
  medications and, 70–71
  shrinking of tissues of, 36
  testosterone levels and atrophy of,
    114–115
  vasocongestion in, 11
genital warts, 89
ginseng, 130
girls, *see* females
GnRH (gonadotropic releasing hormone) an-
    alogs, 65–66
Gräfenberg, Ernst, 15
Graves' disease, 76
growth hormone, 24
G spot, 15
guanethedine, 70
guilt, 47
Gyne-Moistrin, 137

hair
  excessive growth of, 26, 70, 105, 109–110,
    120, 124
  loss, 36, 81, 117, 124
HDL (high density lipoprotein), 110, 111,
    126
headaches, 36, 64–65
heart attacks:

male erectile dysfunction and, 95–96
  sex-induced, 74
heart disease, *see* cardiovascular disease
heart rate during orgasm, 12
herbs, 131–133
heroin, 72
high blood pressure, *see* hypertension
high density lipoprotein (HDL), 110, 111,
    126
hirsutism, 26, 70, 105, 109–110, 120, 124
Hite Report, The, 13, 39
homosexual relationships, 158
honey, 131
hormone replacement therapy (HRT), 6, 23,
    34, 35, 64–65, 106, 145
  see also estrogen therapy; testosterone
    therapy
hormones, 2, 5, 24–27
  after childbirth, 29–30
  after hysterectomy, 83
  libido and, 3, 10, 27–36, 50
  male erectile dysfunction and, 96
  in menopause, 31–35
  in menstrual cycle, 28
  obesity and, 54
  in perimenopause, 30–31
  in pregnancy, 27–29
  receptors, 9
  stress and, 49, 51
  weight loss and, 53
hostility, 49
hot flashes, 30, 34, 35, 65, 132
HRT, *see* hormone replacement therapy
HSD (hypoactive sexual desire), 38, 40, 49
human papillomavirus, 89
hydrocortisone ointment, 89
hypertension, 95, 105, 116
  medications for, 70–71, 96, 100
hyperthyroidism, 76
hypoactive sexual desire (HSD), 38, 40, 49
hypothalamus, 9, 25
hypothyroidism, 76
hysterectomy, 64, 83–86
  libido and, 4, 6
  oophorectomy and, 81, 83
  for pelvic prolapse, 78

imipramine, 67
immune suppressors, 108
implants, penile, 99
impotence, *see* erectile dysfunction, in men
I'm Too Young to Get Old: Health Care for
    Women Over Forty (Reichman), 2
incontinence, 77–78
Inderal, 70
infections, painful intercourse and, 88

infertility, 50, 105
infidelity, 21, 50, 58
injection therapy, penile, 98–99
insomnia, *see* sleep disturbances
insulin, 54, 125
    resistance, 106
intensive sex therapy, 154
International Association of Compounding
        Pharmacies, 123
interstitial cystitis, 89
intimacy, lack of, 57, 60
in-vitro fertilization, 50
irritability, 49
irritable bowel syndrome, 89
ISD: Inhibited Sexual Desire (Knopf and
        Seiler), 148

Janus Report on Sexual Behavior, The, 17–21,
        37
Johnson, Virginia E., *see* Masters and
        Johnson

kava kava, 132
Kegel exercises, 138
ketoconazole (Nizoral), 71
Kinsey, Alfred C., 16
Klonopin (clonazepam), 69
Knopf, Jennifer, 148
K-Y Lotion, 137

labia, 11, 14, 90, 114
lactation, 4, 29–30
Ladas, Harold, 15
Laradopa (L-Dopa), 134
laser surgery, 89
LDL (low density lipoprotein), 110, 111, 126
L-Dopa (Laradopa), 134
lethargy, chemotherapy and, 81
Levlen, 63–64
LH (luteinizing hormone), 25, 26, 48, 65
liberals, sexual activity of, 21
libido, 2–3, 9–10
    age factors and, 4
    assessment of, 40–41, 43–44
    birth control pills and, 62–63
    breast surgery and, 86
    chemical attraction and, 58–60
    chemotherapy and, 81–82
    decreased, 37–38, 40
    depression and, 48, 66
    DHEA supplements and, 127
    diabetes and, 73
    eating disorders and, 53
    estrogen therapy and, 4
    fatigue and, 52–53
    hormones and, 3, 10, 27–36, 65

hysterectomy and, 4, 6
    lactation and, 29–30
    lifestyle and, 137–140
    medications and, 43, 62, 65, 67–71
    in menopause, 31–35
    motherhood and, 4, 29–30
    natural variations in, 57–58
    obesity and, 54–55
    pain and, 29, 88
    in perimenopause, 30–31
    physical development and, 9
    postpartum, 29
    power issues and, 57–58
    in pregnancy, 28
    recreational drugs and, 72
    relationship difficulties and, 56–57
    sexual abuse and, 51
    sexually transmitted diseases and, 78–79
    stress and, 49
    testosterone and, 28, 36, 43, 106–107,
        112–113
Lichen Sclerosis et Atrophicus, 92
licorice, 132
lidocaine gel, 89
lifestyle, libido and, 138–140
limbic system, 9
lipid profile, 118–119, 125, 126
lithium, 69, 89
liver:
    cancer, 112
    functioning of, 112, 116, 118–120, 124,
        128
Loestrin, 63
Lo-Ovral, 63, 65
Lopid (gemfibrozil), 71
Lopressor, 70
lorazepam, 69
low density lipoprotein (LDL), 110, 111, 126
LSD, 72
lubricants, vaginal, 137
Lubrin, 137
lumpectomy, 86, 87
lungs, 74, 97
Lupron, 65
lupus, 75, 127
luteinizing hormone (LH), 25, 26, 48, 65
Luvox, 67

male hormones, 14
    birth control pills and, 62–63
    deficiency of, 112–115
    at perimenopause, 31
    in postmenopausal women, 33
    in puberty, 10, 27
    receptors, 9
    synthesis of, 125

male hormones (*cont.*)
 thyroid disease and, 76
 in women, 23–27, 33, 83
 see also DHEA; testosterone
males:
 DHEA levels in, 124–125
 medical side effects in, 61
 reaction to anger by, 57
 sexual disorders in, 40
 stress in, 49
 testosterone and, 28
 zinc requirements of, 139–140
 see also erectile dysfunction, in men
MAO inhibitors, 67, 134
marijuana, 72
marriage:
 counseling for, 58
 divorce, 40, 56, 58
 frequency of intercourse in, 18
 normal, sexual problems in, 40
 relationship difficulties in, 56–57
married vs. single persons, 18, 39
mastectomy, 86, 87
Masters and Johnson, 12, 15, 16, 29
masturbation, 16, 19–20, 27, 75
medications, 5, 61–62, 133–134
 see also side effects, medication; *specific drugs*
medroxyprogesterone acetate (MPA; Provera; Cycrin), 34, 64
memory lapses, 65
men, *see* males
menarche, 24
menopausal zest, 33
menopause, 2, 30
 chemical, 65
 chemotherapy and, 81–82
 depression in, 48–49
 DHEA levels in, 126
 estrogen therapy in, 64
 herbal remedies for, 132, 133
 libido loss in, 31–35
 medical treatments causing, 80
 sexual pain disorders in, 39
 testosterone and, 35, 106, 108, 113–114
 triglyceride levels in, 110
menstrual cycles, 28, 30
 irregular, 105, 134
menstruation, 25, 53
mesoridazine, 68
methyldopa, 70
methyltestosterone, 35, 117, 119, 120, 122, 124
 troches, 82, 84, 115, 119, 120
micronization, 119, 128
migraines, medications for, 69
minerals, 139

Moist Again, 137
moisturizers, vaginal, 137
monophasic birth control pills, 63, 147
mood stabilizers, 69–70
mood swings, 30, 63, 65
motherhood, libido and, 4
MPA (medroxyprogesterone acetate), 34, 64
multiorgasmic women, 13
multiple sclerosis, 76
multivitamins, 139
muscle relaxants, 69
muscles:
 hormones and, 26, 32, 36
 in intercourse, 12–13
Muse Pellet (alprostadil), 99
myrtle, 132

Naprosyn (naproxen), 71
naproxen (Anaprox; Naprosyn), 71
narcotics, 72
National Health and Social Life Survey,
 17–19, 39
National Institutes of Health, 94
National Opinion Research Center, 20
nausea, chemotherapy and, 81
nerve apathy, estrogen and, 32
neurologic conditions, male erectile dysfunction and, 95
neuroma, 29, 90
neurotransmitters, 9, 70, 134
night sweats, 34
nipples, 11, 27, 36, 113
nizatidine (Axid), 71
Nizoral (ketoconazole), 71
Nordette, 63–64
Norinyl, 63
"normal" sexual activity, 17
Norplant implant, 63
nortriptyline, 67
nursing mothers, libido of, 29–30

odors, sexual response and, 135–136
omeprazole (Prilosec), 71
oophorectomy, 81, 83–84
Oprah Winfrey Show, 3–4, 121
oral contraceptives, *see* birth control pills
orgasm, 10, 12–13
 cervix and uterus in, 84
 clitoral vs. vaginal, 14–15
 frequency of, 13, 19
 in paraplegic women, 16
 testosterone and, 36, 107
 uterine changes in, 15
orgasm center, of the brain, 16
orgasmic disorders, 38–39, 40, 146
 medications for, 68, 69, 71

sexual abuse and, 51
Ortho-Cept, 63, 64
OrthoCyclen, 63–64
Ortho-Novum, 63
Ortho-Novum 7-7-7, 63, 64
Ortho Tri-Cyclen, 52, 63
osteoporosis, 54, 65, 108, 115, 139
ovaries, 3–4
    androstendione production by, 26
    antihormones and, 65, 66
    birth control pills and, 62
    cancer of, 4
    chemotherapy and, 81
    cysts of, 81, 92
    DHEA production by, 26
    estrogen production by, 24
    loss of, 36, 80–81, 83–84, 115
    in menopause, 32–33
    polycystic ovarian syndrome, 105–106
    progesterone production by, 25
    in radiation therapy, 81
    stress and activity of, 49
    testosterone production by, 26
    thyroid disease and, 76
Ovcon, 63, 64
overweight, 33, 54–55, 105, 116
Ovral, 63
ovulation, 25, 29, 53, 76
oysters, 129, 139

pain, 29, 39, 88
painful intercourse (dyspareunia), 39, 88–93
    diseases and, 75
    in epileptic women, 76
    in menopausal women, 32
    sexual abuse and, 51
    testosterone levels and, 114–115
panic disorders, 69
paraplegic women, orgasms in, 16
Parkinson's disease, 133–134
Parlodel (bromocriptine), 134
Paxil, 42, 43, 67
PCO (polycystic ovarian syndrome), 105–106, 117
peer groups, pubescent girls and, 10
pelvis:
    adhesions to, 81, 92
    inflammatory disease in, 88
    pathologies of, painful intercourse and, 88
    prolapse of, 78, 85
penis, 14
    Desyrel and, 67
    implants in, 99
    injection therapy for, 98–99
    vacuum constrictive devices for, 99
    see also erectile dysfunction, in men

Pepcid (famotidine), 71
perimenopause, 2, 30–31, 48, 113
Perioactin (cyproheptadine), 68
periurethral glands, 15
permission, for satisfaction of sexual needs, 152
perphenazine, 68
perspiration, 13, 24, 135
pessaries, 78
pharmacies, compounding, 120, 122–123, 128
phenelzine, 67
phentolamine (Vasomax), 133
Phenytoin (Dilantin), 71
pheromones, 9, 135–136
physical development, libido and, 9
physicians, 2, 4–5
    talking with, 144–148
Pill, the, see birth control pills
pituitary gland, 3, 25, 49
    tumors of, 118, 134
plexus of Frankenhauser, 84
PLISSIT, 152–154
PMS (premenstrual syndrome), 28, 30, 42, 43, 64– 65, 133
politics, sexual activity and, 21
polycystic ovarian syndrome (PCO), 105–106, 117
postpartum depression, 29
posttraumatic stress disorder (PTSD), 51
power issues in relationships, 57–58
pregnancy, 28, 116
Premarin, 34, 35, 123
premenstrual dysphoric disorder, 28
premenstrual syndrome (PMS), 28, 30, 42, 43, 64– 65, 133
prepuce, 31
Prilosec (omeprazole), 71
professionals:
    frequency of sexual encounters of, 21
    stress in, 49
progesterone, 25, 48, 65
    receptors for, 9
    therapy, 23, 66, 82
progestin, 34, 63–64, 112
prohormones, 25–26, 125
prolactin, 29, 68, 118, 134
    receptors for, 9
proprionate, 121
prostaglandin, 98, 133
prostate gland, 97, 132
    cancer of, 125
    surgery on, 96, 102
    zinc and, 139
protriptyline, 67

Provera (medroxyprogesterone acetate), 34, 64
Prozac, 67, 146, 147
psychological factors, 9–10
  in male erectile dysfunction, 95
  post-childbirth libido and, 29
  in sexual disorders, 47–55
  testosterone therapy and, 107
  in vaginismus, 91
psychopharmacologist, 68, 154
psychotherapy, see therapy
psychotropic drugs, 49
  see also antipsychotics
PTSD (posttraumatic stress disorder), 51
puberty, 2, 10, 24, 27–28, 107–108
pubic hair, loss of, 36, 106

race, sexual activity and, 21
radiation therapy, 81, 87
raloxifene (Evista), 64
ranitidine (Zantac), 71
rashness, sexuality and, 47
reading material, erotic, 152–153
recreational drugs, see substance abuse
rectocele, 78
relationship difficulties, 56–57
  communication and, 141–144
  lack of chemistry and, 58–60
  male erectile dysfunction and, 95
  painful intercourse and, 88
  power issues and, 57–58
relaxation techniques, 50
religion, sexual activity and, 21, 28
Remifemin (black cohosh), 132
REM sleep, 16, 127
Replens, 137
reserpine, 70
resolution phase in sexual response, 13
retroverted uterus, 92
rheumatoid arthritis, 75, 108
rhinocerous horn, 129
royal jelly, 131

same-sex relationships, 158
sarsaparilla, 132
saw palmetto, 132
scar tissue, pelvic, 81
scent, sexual response and, 135–136
scleroderma, 75
seafood, 129
sedation, 69
sedentary lifestyle, 116
Seiler, Michael, 148
seizures, 69
selective estrogen receptor modulators (SERMs), 64

selective serotonin reuptake inhibitors (SSRIs), 66– 67, 131, 134
self-confidence, 47
self-consciousness, 47, 54
self-esteem, sexual abuse and, 51
semen, 97
sensate focus exercises, 153
SERMs (selective estrogen receptor modulators), 64
serotonin, 48, 62, 66, 68, 134
  chocolate and, 131
sex hormone binding globulin, see SHBG
sex therapy, 43, 148–157
sexual abuse, 51, 88
sexual activity:
  education and, 21
  of liberals, 21
  "normal," 17
  politics and, 21
  race and, 21
  religion and, 21, 28
  of ultraconservatives, 21
  of ultraliberals, 21
  work and, 20
sexual arousal, 10–11, 15–16
  disorders of, 38, 40, 72, 113
  epilepsy and, 76
  power issues and, 57
sexual aversion disorder, 38
sexual desire, see libido
sexual dysfunction, 38–39, 50
  alcohol and, 72
  medications and, 61, 66–67, 69
  sexual abuse and, 51
sexual fantasies, 16, 21, 27
sexual function, assessment of, 40–42, 43–44
sexual gratification, lack of, 56
sexual health checklist, 41, 42
sexual intercourse:
  blood sugar levels and, 73
  after childbirth, 29–30
  frequency of, 18, 21
  incontinence during, 77–78
  pubescent girls and, 10, 27–28
  testosterone and, 27–28, 107
  vaginal lubrication and, 32
  see also painful intercourse
sexually transmitted diseases (STDs), 58, 78–79
sexual pain disorders, 39, 88–93
sexual rash, 11
sexual response:
  alcohol and, 72
  brain and, 16
  chemotherapy and, 81
  after hysterectomy, 85

male aging and, 97
male hormones needed for, 27
stages of, 10–13
testosterone levels and, 31
sexual self schema scale, 54
sexual stimulation, 14, 15
SHBG (sex hormone binding globulin), 27
age factors in levels of, 31
birth control pills and, 62
caffeine and, 72
in menopausal women, 33, 64
side effects, medication, 61–62
of stress-easing drugs, 50
see also specific medications
sildenafil (Viagra), 6, 77, 84, 99–100, 133
single vs. married persons, 18, 39
Sjogrens syndrome, 75
skeletal formation, estrogen and, 24
skin, 11, 26, 36, 65, 106
sleep disturbances, 30, 34, 65, 107, 132
Smell and Taste Treatment and Research
Foundation, 136
smoking, 20, 31, 97, 116, 140
social factors:
libido and, 9
sexuality and, 47
Society for the Scientific Study of Sex,
156
sodium intake, 70
Solvay Pharmaceuticals, 119, 120
Spanish fly, 130
spicy foods, 130
spinal injuries, 77, 100
spironolactone, 70
Spontane (apomorphine), 133
SSRIs (selective serotonin reuptake inhibitors), 66– 67, 131, 134
STDs (sexually transmitted diseases), 58,
78–79
steroids:
abuse of, 96
creams, 92
Story of O, The, 16
stress:
incontinence and, 77
sexual disorders and, 49–50, 95
substance abuse, 51, 72, 96–97, 149
see also drinking
surgery:
male erectile dysfunction and, 96
for painful intercourse, 89–90
see also breasts, surgery and; hysterectomy
sweat, 13, 24, 135
Symmetrel (amantadine), 67
Synarel, 65
systemic lupus erythematosis, 75, 127

Tagamet (cimetidine), 71
tamoxifen, 64, 82
Tegretol, 69, 77
Tenormin, 70
testes, 24, 26, 97
testicular feminization, 24
testosterone, 24
caffeine and levels of, 72
chemotherapy and, 81
creams, 84, 121–122
deficiency of, 3, 35–36, 43, 96, 98, 106,
112–115
depression and, 48
DHEA converted to, 126
drops, 122
estrogen therapy and, 64
excess of, 105–106
gels, 121, 123
half-life of, 118
injections of, 121–122
male aging and, 97
medications and levels of, 62–64, 66,
68–70
in menopause, 32–33, 35
and menstrual cycle, 28
in midlife, 54
natural vs. synthetic, 119
normal levels of, 114, 120, 147
ointments, 3, 43, 84, 92, 115, 121, 123, 147
patches, 98, 120, 122
in perimenopause, 30–31
in puberty, 27–28
stress and, 49
synthetic, 117, 119
tablets and capsules, 122
test for level of, 118
troches, 122
types of, 118–123
weight loss and, 53
in women, 23, 25–27
testosterone therapy, 4–6, 106–108
after breast cancer, 82–83
contraindications for, 116–117
cosmetic concerns with, 109–110
with GnRH analogs, 66
after oopherectomy, 84
for rheumatoid arthritis, 108
side effects of, 109–112
tests needed for, 117–118
tracking system for, 123–124
thalamus, 12
therapy:
for anger, 58
for depression, 48–49
for eating disorders, 54
for obesity, 55

for PTSD-related sexual problems, 51
for relationship difficulties, 57
for sexual attraction problems, 60
for stress and anxiety, 50
see also specific medications and therapies
thioridazine, 68
thorazine, 68
thyroid disease, 76
thyroid-stimulating hormone (TSH), 76, 118
Touch, 137
tranquilizers, 68, 69
transurethral resection of the prostate
  (TURP), 96
trazadone (Desyrel), 67, 135
tricyclic antidepressants, 67–68, 89
trifluoperazine, 68
triglycerides, 110, 111, 126
Tri-Levlen, 63
Tri-Norinyl, 63
triphasic birth control pills, 63–64, 147
Triphasyl, 63
TSH (thyroid-stimulating hormone), 76, 118
TURP (transurethral resection of the prostate), 96

ultraconservatives, sexual activity of, 21
ultraliberals, sexual activity of, 21
urecholine, 68
urethra, 92
Urispas, 78
uterine insuck, 13
uterus, 15–16
  cancer of, 105, 112
  fibroids of, 65, 92
  lining of, 25
  retroverted, 92
  see also hysterectomy

vacuum constrictive devices, penile, 99
vagina, 11–15
  antibiotics and, 71
  deliveries from, 78
  infections of, 88
  lining of, 24, 30
  in puberty, 24
  sensitivity of, 89
  support devices for, 78
  weight loss and atrophy of, 53
vaginal dryness, 32, 93, 114–115
  autoimmune diseases and, 75
  diabetes and, 73
  herbal remedies for, 132
  lubricants and moisturizers for, 137
vaginal estrogen ring, 82, 84, 115
vaginal fluid, 11, 13, 65
  eating disorders and, 54

in menopause, 32, 34
vaginal hysterectomy, 85
vaginal lubrication, 11, 27
  antihistamines and, 71
  birth control pills and, 62
  in sexual arousal disorders, 38
vaginismus, 39, 76, 88, 91
Vagisil, 137
valproic acid (Depakote), 69, 70, 77
Vaseline, 137
vasoactive intestinal peptide (VIP), 11
vasocongestion, sexual arousal and, 11
Vasomax (phentolamine), 133
very low density lipoprotein (VLDL), 110, 111
vestibulitis, 88
vestibulum, 89–90
Viagra (sildenafil), 6, 77, 84, 99–101, 133
VIP (vasoactive intestinal peptide), 11
vitamin A ointment, 89
vitamin D ointment, 89
vitamins, 139
VLDL (very low density lipoprotein), 110, 111
vomeronasal organ (VNO), 135
vulva, 11, 13, 24, 89
  inflammation of, 91–92
vulvodynia, 89

warts, genital, 89
weight gain:
  chemotherapy and, 81
  corticosteroid drugs and, 75
  in midlife, 54–55
  in puberty, 24
weight loss, 55
  hormone levels and, 53
  for hypertension, 70
Wellbutrin (buproprion), 67, 135, 140, 147
wet dreams, 16
Winfrey, Oprah, 3, 4, 121
women, *see* females
work, sexual activity and, 20

XX chromosomes, 24
XY chromosomes, 24

Yale University School of Medicine, 23
yeast infections, 52, 73, 89, 91
Yocon (yohimbine hydrochloride), 131
yohimbine, 67, 131–132
Yohimex (yohimbine hydrochloride), 131

Zantac (ranitidine), 71
zinc, 139–140
Zithromax, 52
Zoloft, 67
Zyban (buproprion), 67, 135, 140, 147